I have known Jim Qualls for a long time, first as a fellow athlete, then through our mutual profession and more importantly, as a close friend and a caring person. In *Take Care of Yourself*, Jim covers many truths about living that we all know are important and in a manner that is vulnerable by way of his own experiences. He helps the reader realize that, *yes*, I can do this. I can hear Jim's voice so clearly, as if we were having a one-on-one conversation.

Deb Kalish
Attorney

Jim Qualls has succeeded as a family man and community leader. In *Take Care of Yourself*, he provides insight from important life lessons. In 2017, Jim unfortunately was diagnosed with cancer. We rapidly got to know each other. In minutes, I realized how focused he was on taking care of himself. He understood that treatment would be challenging, but he wanted to know how treatment would affect his exercise, nutrition, and singing. Jim clearly is not "the worst waste of six feet," but a man who understands the importance of life. Here he writes a down-to-earth "novel" that allows you to better understand yourself, and through this process how to improve your relationship spiritually and with others.

Trevor Feinstein
Oncologist, Piedmont Cancer Institute

In today's fast-paced, stressful world, everyone is looking for answers to calm the mind, center the spirit, balance one's emotions, and strengthen one's overall physical well-being. *Take Care of Yourself* presents a chapter-by-chapter blueprint through relatable personal stories, perspectives, and sound guidelines to "better the odds" that we can in fact take better care of ourselves and find the overall well-being we want. There are no guarantees in life, but if followed, this book will guide one to an improved state of well-being and support by building better relationships with self, others, and one's community. In short, let Jim lead the way!

William Ott
President, PEAC Ventures, Inc.

Jim brings a lifetime of valuable and varied experience to *Take Care of Yourself*, and it shows. Applicable and relevant from beginning to end, the heartwarming stories in this book are chock-full of encouragement and good advice.

Matt Sapp
Pastor, Central Baptist Church, Newnan, Georgia

Jim Qualls writes about living an "intentional" life, what's important and how to choose to spend one's time. In a world that has too many inputs, Jim's essay topics are sure to give great guidance in how not to just float through life, but to get great joy and fulfillment.

Parks W. Avery
Certified Financial Planner®

Take Care of Yourself is the thoughtful advice of one whose family of origin positively impacted him. The family lived on and loved the land and operated a local store. Jim obviously has a firm foundation he seeks to share. The key word in the title is care, and the essays admonish us to care about how we might best thrive not only as individuals but also as world citizens. Faith informs the living and writing as Jim Qualls lives out his advice, "take care of yourself."

Menlia Moss Trammell
Retired English Teacher

We are blessed to have Jim Qualls in our lives. When he visits us at our cattle farm and plops into one of the rockers on our front porch, our worldview automatically goes positive. As we catch up on family news and share in warm conversation, his upbeat attitude just takes over. No problems, frustrations, or bitterness can thrive when Jim is around! This book will allow you to pull up your rocker and get to know the man we love and admire: the kind, compassionate man who authentically wants to help others lead healthy, joy-filled lives. We urge you to take his advice and become your best self!

Rita and David Brown
Retired Farmers

Take Care
of Yourself

Essays for Life

Jim Qualls

© 2020
Published in the United States by Nurturing Faith Inc., Macon GA,
www.nurturingfaith.net.

Library of Congress Cataloging-in-Publication Data is available.

ISBN: 978-1-63528-092-0

Contents

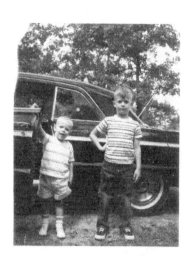

Life nowadays rushes by faster than ever.

Introduction

I was never one of those people, but maybe you were. In high school, they could do seemingly anything athletic and academic. They were popular, promising, and the "Most Likely To." I still admire who they were to some extent. But 20 and 30 and 40 years go by, and things go all sorts of ways.

Some of those overachievers have done exactly that. Some of them have not surprised me at all: they're accomplished, fulfilled, even pillars of the community who are making the world a little better. Others who seemed so promising have fallen on hard times in careers, health, or relationships. Some died robbing a store. Still others who weren't the most beautiful or advantaged have bloomed of their own accord. They look better than ever (maybe we'd just overlooked their beauty back then), they're solid citizens, and they're living happy lives.

George Strait had a hit song titled "She Let Herself Go." That phrase is often uttered after high school reunions. And it's not just her; maybe we guys earn that remark more than the girls do. It's so easy to fall apart in adulthood—and I don't just mean regarding physical appearance.

Life can be cruel. People can be cruel to each other. We can be cruel to ourselves. But it can turn out better than that.

When I was in high school I did pretty well, but I wasn't one of those super athletes or in the Beta Club or in the Alpha Club. I was even told that I was the worst waste of six feet that ever graduated from my high school! I found my own niche, however, through the choral department mainly.

The years went by, and I walked in with my wife at my 20-year reunion. It was fun to see everybody. That was before Facebook, before we could search and lurk and at least scope out our classmates to see how they were doing before the event. I'd been living well away from my hometown and had only seen a handful of classmates since graduation. Nobody knew me as I walked in. I had to introduce myself. It wasn't weight gain so much. I'd lost my hair, gone bald. "Jimmy Qualls? Wow!" But really, I enjoyed the reunion.

Let me make one thing clear that some readers may wonder about: Being "the worst waste of six feet" to ever graduate from my high school never bothered me. I've told that story over and over for years with no pain inside. The guy who said it was a friend, short in stature but a gifted athlete at whatever sport he played. I admired him for that, and, I guess, for at least a second, he thought of what he could do with six feet. I was happy with my niche, my course, my life as it played out, my selfhood. I still am.

Not everyone can say that. That's part of why many of us "let ourselves go." Living daily with gnawing dissatisfactions within takes a toll. Making a living, raising a family, dealing with distractions and troubles and things we do to ourselves and that others do to us can add up.

So, everything I wish to share in this book comes down to this simple phrase, one simple exhortation I'll repeat often: Take care of yourself.

*****

Obviously, there are reasons why I want you to read about taking care of yourself. It's because it matters to me. It's because I see people who have largely avoidable problems. It's because of the people who've inspired me. It's because I've faced some challenges and successes in self-care in my own life.

There are numerous aspects to taking care of yourself. It's not just about one thing or another. I don't claim to be an expert, but I've learned some things that I want to share with you. There's more than what I'll say here, so it won't be exhaustive on any particular subject and I hopefully won't subject you to exhaustion. I hope this all helps you.

*****

Who's got time to take care of themselves? The rush of life is like a kayak in a stream. You have launched into the stream, and life nowadays rushes by faster than ever. You may or may not be aware of the speed of the current. It gets away from most people. Unless you are aware and intentionally navigate, life will get away from you. Today you're 25; tomorrow you're 50. You wake up and wonder how that happened. I hear it all the time. I thought it was just something people said when older people told me life flies by. It's true.

Make your life the best it can be by living right now in the healthiest way possible—healthy in every sense of the word. Don't tell yourself you'll do it later. Don't let anyone lead you into lifestyle choices that are unhealthy.

Take care of yourself in every way now.

*****

I was born into a much slower and quieter world. The year 1961 was much faster and louder than 1928 when my parents were born, but compared to today, it was very different. There were millions less people, millions fewer cars and homes and fast food restaurants. There were no video games, no portable devices by which to play music in your ears, and certainly no phones without cords in your hands. It was just a different world than now.

How we played as children was very different from today, especially for me being fortunate enough to grow up in a very rural place. Nowadays, children have to be little geniuses and super athletes by the time they're six. Stop and think about the children you know and all their involvements. Many parents run themselves ragged making it all happen.

We run through middle school and high school and into early adulthood at a furious pace. I marvel at teenagers with their long daily schedules. I want them to have more time in their lives. Between a full day at school and a load of often endless homework while also being involved in a myriad of activities, the offerings and pressure from adults to keep saying yes to yet another activity seemingly have no limit.

Much of this busyness comes from adults anxiously repeating that we must keep kids busy to keep them out of trouble. Being choosy and thoughtful about it all rarely gets considered. Parents long for more family time together, yet many, even most, jump on the merry-go-round of out-of-control activity. There is precious little opportunity to keep balance.

Author Bill Donahue, in an August 2018 article in *Outside* magazine, wrote about his Catholic cleric uncle who moved to a little French village to live a simpler life. Donahue said, "Very few people are able to transcend the rat race with sustained elegance." So, what will we do? Or, will we just be done unto by time, society, stress, and the elements? It's up to us.

*****

I've always heard people speak of the inevitability of decline—physically, mentally, spiritually, relationally. I've listened countless times as they've told me how it would happen and that getting old is not for sissies and is not fun. I understand much of this, as I've seen older people battle some inevitables. I've been involved with and helped care for older people who've certainly and understandably felt worn and defeated by physical and other difficulties. Those battles are not fun.

I've watched many of those older people over the course of more than 50 years. I realize that some of the things we face are beyond our control, some are of our own doing, and some are because we could have done better. More importantly, there are things we could and should be doing to help ourselves and to help all of us. Some decline is not inevitable. Some of it is inexplicable. Some of it seems cruel. But we can better our odds.

*****

Many of us hope we could just die in peaceful sleep at a ripe old age. Others say they hope they die doing some fun, favorite thing. I've declared that I hope to be found 95 and toothless behind my barn in the mountains of Georgia on a cold, crisp winter day. My wife says I won't be toothless!

Life has proven to me that we don't know the physical challenges we will face. But I must say how I am inspired to do better to take care of myself. First, the more I learn about health, and as findings are challenged and confirmed, the better I can do. And, I am inspired by people who are taking care of themselves physically at all ages, but especially the older they are. I want to be like them: I hope you do, too. By taking care of ourselves physically, the better are our odds as time passes. The benefits are well documented, and more so all the time.

Take care of yourself.

*****

There are people who've always been in my life, whom I've known and loved, who are now facing various types of mental decline. It's tough to see. I also see others who are not nearly as old and wonder what they're doing with themselves. I see people who cannot seem to find their way out of a wet paper bag. I see people who seem to be wasting their lives away, and sometimes wasting my time as they do. Quite often they'll say that's what's happening.

This is not to say anything about people with mental handicaps, who deserve our most compassionate responses. In fact, I would emphatically say that whether mentally handicapped or not, all people deserve compassion.

I wish to focus on what most of us can do to foster our mental and emotional health. What can we do to better our odds mentally and emotionally?

I'm inspired by people older than I am who, even in retirement and later years, have so much on the ball. Whenever I see them, I pay attention and try to emulate their wise, timeless, vibrant ways.

I'm inspired by young people who've wasted no time getting on a healthy track, who've learned to read and hunger for knowledge and truth. They've set out with an orientation that, if they'll keep to it, it will benefit them.

I'm inspired by middle-aged people like me who still have a lot of living ahead and haven't checked out already. I've also been inspired, or motivated, by people I've encountered who've sadly died inside way too early.

There are so many means for turning to anger, sarcasm. selfishness, negativity, and "stuck-ness." We can feast on these things for many reasons. We can in turn make it much worse by abusing alcohol and drugs—and I would add food, hatred, self-hate, abusive relationships, patterns of "drama," and on and on.

On the other hand, thankfully, there are healthy, freeing ways to choose and emulate. It's important to seek out, understand, and incorporate healthy ways into our life—the sooner, the better.

Take care of yourself.

*****

I saw it play out in front of my eyes even in my childhood—people in my life who crashed and burned. I learned early that not everybody loved each other at home, at church, in the neighborhood, in society, or in a war-torn world. Men told me authoritatively as they sipped coffee at my dad's store that relationships would usually sour. They didn't use the word relationships, but they told me it just apparently had to be. Their pontifications were full of sarcasm, as the pain they'd experienced colored the way they saw the world.

For a kid who would have told you in second grade that he wanted to be a wolf biologist, I've instead spent more than 40 years working with people. College education, graduate studies, continuing ed, and "people jobs" all these years have given me a front-row seat on the all-too-common heartache of relational decline.

North of 50 years old now, I can authoritatively say that I've never bought into the inevitability of relational decline. Sarcasm just isn't a steady diet for me: I've seen what such a diet has done to maybe even much of our population.

Take care of yourself.

*****

It's easy to get jaded in this life. Don't let it happen. Ours is a divided era. I can't walk into work or church or a civic or family gathering without being immediately aware that there are different, even polarized, perspectives around the room. While I've developed my own opinions on many things, I'm quite certain my methods for developing these opinions have evolved. I want to be more objective and considerate than I've ever been, because more than ever I believe "the truth will set you free." And, so, I cannot let sarcasm and bitterness and prejudice tell me that everything inevitably will go downhill. Some things are better. Some things need fixing.

I've always been involved in bringing hope to our world. An initial little boy's wish to be a wolf biologist has turned into a lifelong in-depth study of our natural world and involvement in environmental conservation, even though I missed a turn and didn't quite make it onto *Wild Kingdom*. And, all these years of "people work" haven't soured me. Instead, I'm more sure than ever that with one word, one deed at a time, we can do the better thing in our society and our world. It's not "dog eat dog." In taking care of those around us, we in turn take care of ourselves.

Take care of yourself without being selfish.

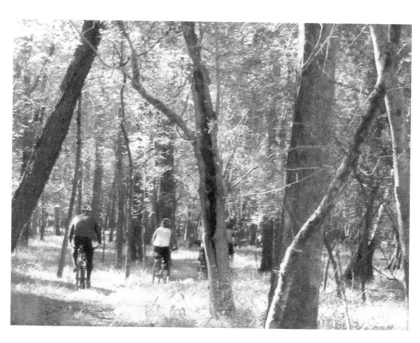

No matter what is going on in your life right now,
take care of your body.

Chapter 1

Take Care of Your Body

The mere mention of "take care of yourself" elicits from most people that, "OK, we're gonna talk about fitness and eating right and exercise." So, let's do just that.

Would you agree that there's more said about fitness than ever before? Would you agree that there's yet more need to talk about fitness? Would you agree that many people need to shape up? Would you say you are as fit as you should be or could be or want to be? If not, why?

Do you know how many times I've asked myself these questions? Do you know how many times I haven't liked the answer? For your best interests, plow ahead to dig into the idea of taking care of your body. No matter how you've been doing, no matter your age, no matter what is going on in your life, start improving how you take care of your body.

A healthy body is an important investment. It is at least as important as whatever financial investments you are making or need to make. So, do it. There's no better time than now. Time will pass anyway, so spend it taking better care of your body. It's not about vanity or self-image; it's about being the best you can be both now and in the future.

Health and fitness are important to me, but it hasn't always been that way. I grew up in a family where it was rarely ever mentioned or a priority. That's the way it was for most families we knew in that era. We didn't exercise, run, walk, or work out, and few people we knew other than high school athletes ever did. Our family had emerged from an agricultural economy, and, aside from our manual labor in farming and at our home place, we didn't work out. We did eat lots of fresh vegetables from our sizable home garden, however.

When I was 10 years old, my dad made a career change and bought what was then a country store just down the road from our home. He dove right in and started working 14-hour days, making a go of the business. He succeeded for 21 years.

My hometown flipped the switch into hot growth mode just as my dad bought the store. None of us had seen that coming, but the timing was very fortunate. The business evolved quickly from a sleepy country store in the heart of what had been an idyllic rural community to a busy convenience store that yet maintained a country store feel. People loved it and gave my dad a loyal following.

I started working at the store immediately, helping whenever I could. And everything in front of me was free for the taking. I had all the Cokes, chips, ice cream, cinnamon rolls, candy bars, sandwiches, burgers, pizzas, and more that I wanted.

I remember our pediatrician warning my brother and me to lose some weight. Growth spurts and high school helped us some, but I have struggled with the American diet with varied success throughout the years. Thankfully, I've gradually won more and more. You can either "win the war" or give in and just let yourself go. Either way, there's a price to pay.

For most Americans today, when it comes to eating the wrong things and weight gain and lack of fitness, it's easy to get caught up in what seems inevitable and unavoidable. Most of us speak of it in just those terms. Reality is different, however. It would be wonderful if we could just snap out of this mindset. I insist it is indeed possible, although many of us resign ourselves to it while others of us just don't care. But there comes a day, sooner or later, that reality smacks us in the face. When that happens, we wish we hadn't given in, hadn't let ourselves go, had done something about it. It would be better for a host of reasons if we had started taking care of ourselves earlier.

I chose to do something about my situation. My first efforts in high school in the 1970s were mainly fueled by girls. I reckoned that girls would like me better if I wasn't a walking result of all that stuff I ate at my dad's store. I wasn't ever athletic. My only foray into athletics was Little League Baseball in my third and fourth grade seasons. I showed absolutely no promise as a baseball player. I just wanted to go back home and be on the farm. In fact, in high school, as I rapidly shot up past 6 feet tall, I turned down a couple of recruiting efforts from the football team (and succeeded instead in the choral music department). I cannot say I mastered health and fitness practices in those days, but I at least managed to shed being overweight.

In college I gradually improved my diet just a little and even took up efforts at exercising. I'd do push-ups in my dorm room, ride a bike around campus, or walk around town. Also, several health crises of some people in my life gave me early exposure to the need to behave better. So, that spurred me on. Into my 20s and 30s I kept all that up with varied success and failure, but increasingly I won the victories.

Many of us talk a lot about fitness but get no further. It's easier to just talk about fitness or exercise or eating better than it is to do it. We can get into a rut of being fitness spectators or "wannabes" only. And we buy all kind of fitness paraphernalia but never do what it takes to get fit. I've done my share of all this, but I'm thankful I moved on to take action and develop habits of actively pursuing fitness.

Treadmills and stationary bikes were not meant to become clothes racks. My old Hamsterbike has close to 15,000 miles on it, even though I don't really like it! Times of inclement weather and difficult schedules and circumstances have made it handy for me to at least maintain fitness and keep up the fitness habit. Though I always crave my real bike, my Hamsterbike has proven a good investment.

Some folks can tell you about every low-fat product on the middle aisles of the grocery store, yet never venture near the outer aisles where the produce and other less processed foods are found. They can tell you all kinds of calorie counts, or how much weight they've lost this time or need to lose. I remember a couple of my teachers in the 60s and 70s who drank Tab fat-free soft drinks and ate potato chips. They were the first people I remember talking about dieting. Yet I also have childhood memories of how that strategy wasn't working.

There's still way too much spending on artificial means for chasing fitness. Even so, it's great to see at least larger numbers of people gravitating to natural eating habits and to effective exercise habits. "Eating closer to the tree" and pursuing fitness practices that you'll keep doing are just two that I want to emphasize here.

Too often, we talk about fitness "too little too late." I've seen it countless times. Someone gets a symptom or something unexpected gets detected at a doctor visit. The doctor prescribes, among other things, an immediate healthy lifestyle: eating healthier and getting regular exercise. But what the doctor specifies and what the patient "hears" may vary greatly. Countless patients have gone from that key moment and made a temporary and halfhearted effort at healthier living only to resume their bad habits in a short time.

My own fitness discoveries make me want to do more. The more fit we are, the more "freed" we are to feel good and enjoy the benefits. I've often said that even if I died next week, pursuing fitness makes me feel better for now. Too many of us see this as the last thing we want to do, however. We say we're too busy or we don't have the time or energy or just plain don't want to do it. We talk ourselves out of making the effort, of jumping up from the couch and having a workout for a small fraction of each day. We engage in everything else instead of going out the door and taking a walk or rolling our bike out of the garage and enjoying the "whee" that it offers. There's a whole world beyond the couch and the door that we need to discover and enjoy.

Make discipline a priority.

You may associate discipline with punishment or grueling difficulty or frustrating assignments, but that's not what we're talking about. Discipline can be a good thing; it can help you get what you want. You do want to be more healthy and fit, don't you? Then, turn down the momentary tasty pleasure of the office doughnuts so that you'll be glad you made progress on your health and fitness goals. Plan ahead what you will and won't eat at birthday celebrations and office parties, over the Fourth of July holiday, on vacation, during Labor Day weekend, or at Thanksgiving. (And don't forget about all that Halloween candy after you send your kids to bed.)

Discipline is grabbing some time in each busy day to get in a spin on a stationary bike or take a walk or ride a bike or do a workout because you realize it will all pay off. Discipline is doing now what will benefit you later. It's prioritizing what will help you the most. It's sticking to what ultimately brings you the most joy and pleasure. Discipline is getting in some exercise ahead of social media or screen time or a movie—unless you work out while watching that movie. Learn to like the word discipline. See it as doing something good for you so that everything in life can be better.

For the record, I've had my struggles with fitness through the years. I can refer to times in my life when I was unhappily overweight and unfit. People who've known me a long time often deny remembering me like that, but I do. There are few photos for a reason. I've never qualified as obese, but at times I've certainly been overweight and unfit. It has rarely been in me to laugh at fat people, because, first it's wrong, and second I've usually been aware that it wouldn't take that much for me to be them. I've seen so much of it, and I could just decide to give up and let myself go. I've even thought about it for a minute here and there.

What about you? Not overweight? You may not be off the hook either! There's this term "skinny fat" for folks who are slim or even skinny but are not fit. They have few advantages over those who are fat. They need change, too. (I've had some moments in this category.) Much has been said and written about the needs of people in this category in recent years. Combating it, I love the phrase, "Strong is the new skinny."

In later chapters in this book we'll point out that people can have the fittest physiques but be dead and cold inside. Being honest about ourselves and our habits and choices are first steps to becoming better. But first, we must face the facts. There are many ways to die, and even more ways to live! Facing our realities is the first step toward better living. It's the first step in moving toward what we want to become, even if we haven't put our finger on it yet.

The condition of our population is well documented by observation and by countless books, documentaries, and articles. And, if you watch television even a little, you can quickly count all sorts of offers for weight loss or for styles that will miraculously transform you. Also, compare photos of groups of people today to photos taken in 1961, the year I was born. Now, take a drive around especially fast-growing urban and suburban areas, and watch for the increased presence of varied medical specialty clinics. They service the exponentially growing ailments we are incurring largely due to our lifestyles. That's not to make anyone feel bad about unavoidable maladies, but I know what it makes me want to do: take better care of myself.

A few years ago, it was time to move our younger daughter into a new dorm at Berry College. Everything had to go to the third floor. It was a hot August day. The agreement was that Dad would help with the heavy lifting, then be free to play while all the girly decorating took place. So, after hauling the stuff up, off to play I went.

I unloaded my mountain bike off the car and ground up the gravel road ascending Lavender Mountain. Up there at the House of Dreams, you can see for miles in all directions. I relaxed a bit, watered up, enjoyed the views, then started down the gnarly mountain bike trail, a much more direct route. By gnarly I mean roots and ruts and rocks, so much so that many folks shouldn't attempt to walk it. I made it down with no problem, then found myself on a flat, calm gravel path in the valley.

Making a turn at no more than 10 miles an hour, suddenly my bike went left and I went right, smack down on my face. My right hand went up a small embankment. There was the problem. I rolled over to see how many people were laughing at me, but no one was around. I knew I had some aches, but nothing serious immediately evident. I slowly rolled back to my car, loaded the bike, and went back to the dorm for assessment by my ladies. A sponge bath and pain relievers finished out the day. I was sore on Sunday.

On Monday morning I went to see my long-lost orthopedic surgeon. He diagnosed a dinged right rotator cuff. The main treatment was a month off the bike and minimal movement, hopefully avoiding surgery. He was right and I've been fine ever since, but there's more. When I'd first started the visit with the orthopedist, we recounted my previous visit, with surgery, from a mountain bike crash in 2004 that could have been avoided. I told the doctor how embarrassing this one was: a flat gravel path, going maybe 10 miles per hour. I felt stupid. The good doctor proceeded to tell me what had happened to him recently.

My orthopedist had been working late one night at the hospital and was ready to go home when a summertime thunderstorm came up. He waited and waited. Thinking there was a break in the action, he dashed across the parking lot but tripped over a curb and had to make his way to the emergency room. He asked me, "Does that make you feel better, Jim?" I said, sure it does!

Things can happen to us in ordinary activities. We need to face our realities and limitations yet live so that we have healthy, vibrant, interesting lives. As I'm fond of saying to folks who question my mountain biking and other things I do (while they advocate their sedentary lifestyles), "More people die on the couch than anywhere else."

In an age when health care benefits from science and specialization more than ever, and in the United States where we claim to be the best there is, health care collectively and individually is one of our biggest challenges. A "what's mine is mine" attitude among those of us who have more doesn't help. Too many victims are being created, and we really aren't facing the deep bottom-line cost; instead, we're just yelling at each other about it. Also, how we view health care cries out for change.

If we would work better at prevention, nutrition, exercise and stress management, it would affect our health care scene tremendously. It would make better human and financial sense to deal with these challenges with care and compassion, and at the same time work toward long-term solutions. Many of us also realize additional religious, humanitarian, and ethical reasons that spur us to help those around us achieve better care. It just makes sense.

Invest in prevention and wellness.

Decades ago, largely aided by the commercial effect on our common culture, we became a pill-oriented society. Whatever malady we have, surely there is an instant cure in a pill. Also, the way we viewed and accessed food completely changed. As a result, our food has become less healthy. What once was the norm has become a specialty: organic food. I am thankful for its recovery and continued growth. And, for more and more of us, we have begun to incorporate physical activity into our lives instead of allowing our push-button world to make us so sedentary. Still, most people I know have poor diets and avoid exercise. They don't seem to want it any other way, or else don't make healthy choices.

Health care for most of us amounts to care when we are sick and ailing. We wait to be fixed when we break down instead of building and maintaining good health and enjoying the benefits of it. We need to develop strength as much as possible for the good days and in case of the bad days.

Investing in wellness makes "cents" for individuals and companies and on a national level. It makes sense for now and in the future. It makes long-term, bottom-line financial sense for all involved. You and I should see our bodies as assets, precious possessions that should be maintained even more than we maintain our homes, cars, wardrobes, and whatever else. Do you know people who make wellness that kind of priority? Should you make it top priority?

Wellness includes not only our bodies but also our stress levels and much more—and those other aspects affect our bodies in turn. We should take care of our wellness in all those aspects and not live to regret what we've done to ourselves. Smart companies are realizing that it makes sense to their bottom lines to invest in and facilitate their employees' wellness. Smart nations are doing the same.

Are you taking care of your overall wellness? Does your company offer wellness benefits and provide a healthy and happy atmosphere in which to work? Do some honest research into how the USA is or is not investing in healthcare and wellness versus that of some other nations. See what questions it raises for us all.

Our wellness and prevention practices need refocusing—individually, corporately, and nationally. We need a new perspective, attitude, and prioritization. For too many of us, our jobs and related stress are killing us. Add in the personal drama so common in our lives and it's a wonder we do as well as we do. I've seen the "drama" in the lives of people at home, in traffic, at church, at school, in the neighborhood, at civic clubs and community organizations, and on and on. We need an awakening to the drama we're creating in all these aspects of life—and then work toward eliminating it. (Personally, if you bring drama my way, I'll deal with you first and then avoid you.)

While seeking to take care of ourselves and better our odds, we also need to care about the health of others. Health care is a political football game that we must win for all. Let's not be part of the problem, politically or personally, so that we can better our odds of not needing as much healthcare and of recovering better when we do.

Clean up your diet.

I love to eat! My appetite has always been a little too good. I'm not a foodie per se, but I do enjoy good food. What are my favorites? If I didn't care, I'd eat cheeseburgers three times a day—good ones, because life is too short for mediocre cheeseburgers. Cheeseburgers have always been my default request. When I was growing up, after appointments with my pediatrician in downtown Atlanta, my folks would take me to the Varsity for those famous hamburgers.

In the 1960s my dad managed a ranch in Roswell, Georgia, that hosted rodeos. I accompanied him a lot, and he would turn me loose with five dollars. Back then I could have all the burgers and colas I wanted with that amount of money—and I did. It was mediocre rodeo food, but I remember finding it tasty. These days I have my choices, so I try to stick to truly good burgers—even though I enjoy steak.

There's something else I'm a little famous for: chips. If I get a hold of a bag, no matter the size, I'll probably empty it. So, more and more I do not bring chips home. I still enjoy a little bag when eating out at lunch sometimes, with barbeque chips being my long-time favorites.

I also love biscuits, cornbread, country-fried steak, pizza, and all sorts of stuff. Ever since helping my dad open his store at 6:30 a.m. when I was out of school, I have loved sausage biscuits. I would heat up some sausage biscuits, grab a V8, and crawl up on the ice machine out front to watch the sunrise. The store faced east, so there it was, and there I was.

I love desserts, too. I love good cinnamon rolls and my wife's famous apple pie. I love Blue Bunny ice cream sandwiches. I love rich moist cakes, especially old-fashioned chocolate or fudge cakes, caramel cakes, and my wife's rendition of the Betty Crocker apple spice cake. And I can hardly resist my daughter's wonderful homemade cupcakes. Then there are Snickers bars and Oreo cookies and Dairy Queen blizzards.

Over the last several years I've dialed down my sugar intake considerably, based on what I kept reading about sugar and also due to how I observed it made me feel: less sugar = better; more sugar = worse. Add to that what I have discovered about the connection between sugar and cancer and most common diseases. Less sugar has meant a fitter, leaner body for me. My sugar intake is now at the lowest ever in my life.

Before I stop to analyze, let me also say I've always been a huge fan of farm-grown, garden-fresh foods. Since I was a kid, I've said just give me some fresh crowder peas and cornbread and I'll be very satisfied. And, there's creamed corn, especially from my favorite restaurant on the earth, the world-famous Dillard House. But there's a huge list of vegetables I enjoy and always will.

Oh, I've eaten some bad stuff! I hope my body will forgive me. North of 55 years old, I'm cognizant that I want to make up for all that as much as I can muster. Especially when I reflect back on the artificial, chemical-laden foods I've taken in, it makes me shudder. So, at this half of life, I'm really trying to make up for the previous years by majoring on what is truly healthy. It takes a little learning and constant determination, but it's freeing and rewarding to eat better and feel better.

Most of us need to seriously clean up our diets. Just look at us, at what we eat, at what it's doing to us. When you study chronic illness, childhood obesity, pregnancy difficulties, early onset diseases such as diabetes, joint maladies, and on and on, you realize much of it has to do with our dietary choices and lifestyles. No, not everything can be prevented, but much of it could be.

I've been telling folks for years that even if I die next week, for now, I'll feel better by taking care of myself and eating better—and maybe I even look a little better. I definitely sleep better, move better, have more energy, am more creative, sing better, and have better health stats when I eat properly. On the other hand, no matter how fun some indulgences seem at the time, if strung out in succession, I do not feel well. We need to take pride in and care for ourselves because it will make us happier than stuffing ourselves full of pizza night after night.

Healthy eating can be good eating. Many people think healthy eating is iceberg lettuce salads and bad eating is bacon. That's not true. It's possible to get a variety of tasty, fresh ingredients and to incorporate them into a repertoire of healthy and enjoyable eating. Healthy eating also involves avoiding a hurried pace. I try to take time to pause for a breath, some thought, some thanks. And, I enjoy mealtime connections with others. I'm always truly more thankful after I've eaten, reflecting on the goodness I enjoy while remembering that some people live in a "food desert" and / or do not have "a place at the table."

Eat close to the tree.

A phrase I've latched on to the last few years is that of "eating closer to the tree." That means eating simpler and more natural ingredients. I've also incorporated another motto: If you can't spell it or pronounce it, don't eat it. This comes to mind when we examine the ingredients list of many of our favorite foods, of many items on store shelves, especially on the inner aisles of grocery stores. The fewer the ingredients, the simpler. The more natural, and, yes, the more "spell-able" and "pronounce-able" they are, generally the better. So, name your fruits or vegetables or meats; add butter (genuine, unadulterated, preferably organic free-range, local butter) and other simple ingredients and spices; and enjoy!

So, what's the magic with simpler ingredients? Why do they matter? What are the benefits? I don't mean to say that everything we eat should have no more than three ingredients. In fact, the incorporation of a variety of foods—and as my mother-in-law would emphasize, a variety of colors—is always better.

But what I am saying is that each ingredient can and should be natural and healthy. It's simply how we're meant to eat: real food, not food-like products. The health benefits matter.

In addition to how pleasurable healthy eating can taste, I've found it goes down easier, stays down better, and the way I feel after I eat is greatly improved. So, immediately there are multiple, exponential benefits. Every time I go with the healthier choices, I'm immediately glad due to how I feel and, I'll venture to say, how I look. (Okay, forget the looks thing; let's just emphasize that clothes fit and feel better.) And that's just the beginning.

Think of food as fuel.

While some people invest in fitness by working out a lot or doing a lot of aerobic exercise, they still struggle with weight. Their diet is obviously a problem. We need to think of food as fuel for our body, rather than as filling a temporary want or need. We need to be truthful with ourselves about what and how we eat.

Admit that you're ordering pizza too often, that you indulge too often in desserts, that you overeat or undereat, that you grab a bag of chips at night and munch away to deal with boredom or anxiety. Be kind to yourself, but face whatever is handicapping and sabotaging you. We have to clean up our diets. Over time and with consistency, we'll see the changes we want that can last a lifetime.

Since way back, I've heard people say about food: "It all goes to the same place." They were talking about the odd combinations of foods they typically "wolfed" down together. My dad was one of those folks. After a hard day's work, he'd sit down at the table and pile all his food together. All food does go to the same place, and it's meant to be fuel for our body. It matters what we take in.

If you pulled up at a gas station and you knew there was water or sugar in the gas, would you fill up? Of course not! You care about your car. Why would you fuel your body with so much bad stuff? Your body is your most precious possession so give it utmost care in what you feed it. I understand the fun of "recreational eating" and indulgences we all tend to enjoy, but we should recognize that most of us overindulge too often and with regularity, and it's causing us multitudes of problems.

Practice healthy eating habits.

My wife and I have had a good arrangement for 35 years in that I'm a good food "obtainer" and my wife is a wonderful cook. We don't generally have time to linger in the kitchen, but I've always been thankful for what our family has shared and enjoyed there. Yeah, we watch our share of food channel shows, sometimes while we're eating at our kitchen island, but we're not exactly foodies. However, good things have been happening in recent years when it comes to cooking at home and how we approach eating. More and more people are combining artful cooking with healthy eating. Also, the farm-to-table and locally grown movements have been the best thing to happen to food and eating in decades.

Farm to table, locally grown, organically grown, free-range, grass-fed, and the like are better for all of us and our environment. They're worth our investments of a few more dollars if for nothing else than the increased nutritional value. At our home we've noted how we've benefited by not buying indulgent, junk food items and instead spending that money on healthier, organic, local-type foods. It's easy logic. Drop the desserts, the boxes of snack items, the sugary drinks, and spend that same money on higher quality foods that give increased health benefits. And, I tell folks all the time how much better organic fruits and vegetables and grass-fed milk and other foods I eat taste versus the other stuff.

Healthy eating is doable, but it's tougher if you're in a "food desert." It can be difficult to eat healthy at every meal, especially if work schedules and logistics follow certain patterns. It's easier if you work from home and can stock the refrigerator and pantry with tasty, healthy foods or if you work somewhere set up for employees to bring, store, and heat up lunches and snacks. But if you're on the move with your job, as I have been over many years, you must scope things out and make the healthiest choices possible—often in a hurry. It can be tough, depending on where you find yourself, especially in a "food desert." But wherever you are, make the effort to find the healthiest food choices.

I cannot say enough about how much eating healthier has helped me. Now, for those people who know me well, who've joined me for meals that were less than pristine, I'll admit that those weren't healthy. But they were fun! Maybe it was a family gathering, a getaway to the North Georgia mountains, or some other gathering where we indulged. Nobody likes that better than

I do, but it's not an everyday thing. I've also thoughtfully and intentionally moved to doing less and less "recreational eating" and largely cut out sugars from my diet—especially desserts, candy bars, and good ole sweet tea (I now drink it with honey or unsweetened tea).

All these changes have helped me reduce pounds and increase leanness. It feels much better being leaner: I'm just more comfortable and have more energy and endurance. Cleaning up my diet has helped improve my blood levels of items such as triglycerides. Eating cleaner helps me decrease reflux problems, vocal and upper respiratory troubles, and helps me sleep better and longer.

When you're a 15-year-old kid and running cross country and growing at the same time and then scarfing down pizza at night, it seems to work out. You seem to get away with eating crazy. It's fun! I did my share of it. But then you go off to college and you hear about the "freshman 15"—15 extra pounds that suddenly appear in the first semester or two. Then it keeps on going up from there. Fast forward to your late 20s or early 30s—maybe blame it on marriage or work—and then to your 40s and 50s and it's time to clean up your diet. It's possible, one day at a home, one choice at a time, to eat cleaner than ever. Some people succeed at eating cleaner by planning their meals weekly. I encourage you to do that.

Stock up on salads, fruits, vegetables, and proteins.

In the past I really wasn't a salad and fruit person. Let's go right to the meat and potatoes! In the past three years especially, I've eaten more salads and fruit than probably in all my life combined. And I'm still ratcheting up my intake. Color helps with nutritional value and also with taste and appeal. So, get more variety; eat more colors.

Now, about the veggies. I was a lucky boy. I grew up on a farm where we had our own garden, our friends and neighbors had gardens, and our relatives had gardens. From an early age I loved the smell of the freshly plowed Georgia red clay in our garden. Our whole family helped plant, tend, and harvest the garden. It was probably a quarter of an acre. We'd plant seeds and, in my eagerness, a few days later I'd go scratch down a little bit and see the beans sprouting and heading to the surface. I enjoyed cutting up "seed potatoes" and watching them sprout up. I loved seeing the corn and okra and peas emerge from the soil. I still love the smell of a pea patch, fresh-cut okra, and freshly shucked corn.

From those experiences as a kid, I also learned to love the taste of many, though not all, vegetables. (There's some I still don't like.) Since when I was maybe seven years old, folks have heard me say crowder peas and cornbread are two of my favorite things. And I'm nuts about fresh creamed corn—especially Silver Queen corn—and, like the cornbread, not sweetened. (Don't ruin it: Leave it unadulterated, the way it was meant to be.)

Discover the variety of vegetables out there, try to get them locally or grow them yourself, and make them a regular part of your diet and lifestyle. The same is true of fruits: Increase the amount, add more variety and colors, and obtain those grown locally and organic. In fact, some people are wisely calling fruit the new fast food, because it can be obtained at various places, needs no cooking, and is portable. Eating fruits and vegetables is how people have lived and improved their health through the millennia, and we're getting wiser by rediscovering it.

Then there are proteins. First, let's talk about meats. I've been involved in animal agriculture all my life. I know it and love it. Just as I turned three years old in 1964, we moved to Roswell, Georgia, where my dad managed a horse and cattle ranch for much of a decade. From that time until just before my folks sold our place in 1999, we also had cattle of our own. Sometimes it was just a couple; sometimes it was upwards of 20. Though I've spent much time in suburbia, I've kept my head, heart, and hands in the cattle business. I've read continuously, attended cattle events multiple times per year, and, for a number of years now, I've been fortunate enough to have dear friends nearby who have a 425-acre, grass-fed cattle ranch. I visit with them for fun and friendship, but we always check the cattle together, discuss cattle husbandry and breeding, and I help them with various care tasks with the cattle.

I understand the post–World War II grain-fed cattle industry. I don't blame people in it unfairly, but I've become more and more convinced of the disadvantages and detriments of that relatively short-term practice. I am convinced of the present and future benefits of sustainable practices in animal agriculture, benefits to our environment, the animals themselves, and to us the consumers. For our purposes here, though, I'll focus on the nutritional benefits of sustainably raised meat.

They have better nutrition and taste, with increased omega-3s versus less desirable meats. So, at our home, we are consuming more grass-fed beef, organic chicken and the like, plus patronizing more restaurants that feature grass-fed beef, free-range chicken, and even other local meats on their menu. People are flocking to these places. It is the future, and yet it is the past. And, it is indeed healthier for you and me. White Oak Pastures in Bluffton, Georgia calls it "radically traditional farming." Look them up online and on social media and in your grocer's meat case.

In addition to meat, there are other proteins. Ok, I'm nuts about peanut butter! I've always liked it. Years ago, I switched to fully natural peanut butter—just peanuts and salt. I open the jar, stir up the contents with a knife, and then put it in the refrigerator. There it sets up and the oil quits rising to the top. Peanut butter plus milk (preferably organic, grass-fed) offer a double shot of protein. Another protein source for me is spinach (like Popeye, I "eats me" spinach), which offers multiple health benefits.

As I've indicated, buying local meat and produce matters. I understand if your thought of obtaining food is one weekly stop at one grocery store, but even that is improving as grocery stores are featuring locally grown products. There are nutritional benefits that come from locally grown, in addition to the freshness factor. Also, such as in local honey, many people advocate that there are health benefits that come from honey from bees that have been visiting local flowers. Local foods require less fuel and pollution in their production and distribution. And, eating local foods supports local economies. It helps to know where your food originates. So, when you see some of us reading labels in the grocery store or farmers markets, we're not just looking at nutritional stats: we're looking at where it comes from.

Practice mindful eating.

If every time we get ready to eat, we would pause a second to think, "How will this make me feel?" our choices would improve. This habit has helped me so much. When I began realizing, for example, that ice cream in the evening would wake me up at 3 a.m., I began to learn. When I began to be aware how much my habit of destressing at night by killing a box of Cheez-Its or a bag of barbeque potato chips was causing weight gain and acid reflux, I had to make changes. When I began to grasp the importance of what I "fuel" my body with, I began to "fuel up" with foods that would make me feel better.

When I sit down in a restaurant these days and look at the menu, indulgences still jump off the page at me. But I've gained the wisdom to more often move on to find the healthier items that I also like and that I'll be glad two hours later that I've chosen. It's not just knowing I made healthier choices that makes me feel good, but actually how those foods make me feel. Doing that day after day and over time, the satisfaction grows.

Let's say it's Thanksgiving week/season/month. There's the office party, the church dinner, the neighborhood dinner, and a couple of family dinners because not everybody can make it on Thanksgiving Day. Before you know it, one day of indulgence turns into way too many days. All that wonderful food and everybody's creations can taste so good, but it adds up. I love all that as much as anybody, but I've realized I have to eat so that I won't regret it. I've learned to artfully dodge my way through the food land mines at times such as these and make choices I won't regret. I've simply had to back off and ease up on my eating.

Eat to fight decline.

We tend to use the word "decline" to describe elderly people who are noticeably losing health. Actually, decline starts early in life—even in our 20s and 30s. Decline doesn't have to be inevitable and can be reversible; it's something we can control to an extent. For all those who are dealing with the freshman 15 and beyond, this is your call. Do something now! Now that I'm in my mid-50s, I have seen enough to say: Get going now, do yourself a favor, and eat in ways that you'll live to be glad about. Break out of the bad habits you've started and discover the good stuff. Build stock in your health just as we talk about building financial stocks from an early age.

Eating leaner can fight decline. This isn't about losing weight or being slim; you can be skinny but very unhealthy. Eating to be leaner helps with longevity, frees you to move and feel better every day, and brings added health benefits both now and in the long term. (Clothes also fit better.)

While eating to fight decline, don't overlook the importance of proper hydration. Between half and three fourths of us at any time are at least mildly dehydrated. We need to drink more. I've developed a habit of downing a glass of water as soon as possible after I get up every morning. Drinking throughout the day just makes everything go better! Being hydrated helps with energy and endurance and aids digestion. Hydration is important before, during, and after exercise and can also help avoid headaches. I've also found hydration to be helpful to me as a singer.

Water is best for hydration. There are many things folks are guzzling that do the opposite of hydrating: they act as stimulants, dehydrate as diuretics, and contain unneeded sugars that drag us down. Good, clean water is so important for you and me.

Kick the sugar habit.

Perhaps nothing I can say about health and fitness could be more important than urging readers to kick our society's sugar habit. It's long been a problem, but recent decades have seen the abuse of sugar increase exponentially. It's everywhere and in everybody's hands. We must become aware of how much sugar we're consuming and where it's found. And we need to become aware of the multitude of problems it's causing for us. No dietary change I've made has helped me more than cutting down on sugars. And, yes, a host of common diseases center around our sugar habit, so cutting sugar helps reduce those problems. I love cake and pie and ice cream and sweet tea and many other things, but the more I give them up, the less I regret it. I just feel better, and yes it helps me get leaner. So, I urge you to:

• Identify the sugars you're consuming.
• Realize that once the moment of pleasure in the mouth is over, the good feeling is over.
• Cut down on or cut out altogether cake, pie, candy, sports drinks, soft drinks, and other sugary foods and drinks.
• Focus on the healthier you that you want to become.
• Think about what you have to lose if you keep consuming too much sugar.
• Think about what you have to gain if you get your sugar habit under control.

Get adequate sleep.

I've been guilty over much of my adulthood of not getting enough sleep. I'm a night owl who's had to operate on everybody else's time, meaning early to rise but also staying up late. Thankfully, I rarely have trouble sleeping. But as time has gone on, I've had to "invest in more rest." How about you? Are you getting enough sleep? Coffee and stimulants aside, how does it go for you? Studies show that most of us don't get enough good sleep.

It can be crazy these days! Schedules run all over the place, or people just throw out schedules and go nuts. And then there are all the expectations from "the authorities" at work, at school, and wherever else that matters. So, we burn the candle at both ends, run ourselves to exhaustion, and often become blind to what we're doing. Or, we know we're exhausted and out of steam but can't find a place to jump off. The arrival and widespread use of the light bulb may be partly to blame.

With the discovery of electricity came an artificial extension of the day. Prior to that time, in a more agrarian society, most people worked from sunup to sundown, and even some on either side of those limits. The light bulb isn't going away any time soon. We have countless "cities that never sleep." And some of us almost never sleep. (I've seen my share of workdays that started before daylight and ended way after daylight.) Lack of sleep compromises our health and robs us of personal time, causing some people to lament that they "don't have a life." It cannot be sustained indefinitely.

Work schedules are also part of the problem with sleep. Many hardworking people hardly get home before they have to turn around and go back to work. Or, some have jobs where they are always "on call," and they get called back out again. Or, maybe they get to go home, but someone is constantly calling or texting them at odd hours with some question or "crisis." Sometimes we pass it off as the price of success. Smart employers are realizing that to keep good employees, they must make their work lives sustainable, doable, and even desirable. They realize the cost of turnover and so, in turn, want to help avoid burnout. Over time, it pays them to do so.

Avoid always being "on."

Even before the advent of the cell phone, I served in jobs where I was "always on." The cell phone and texting and changes in professional practices have eroded "closing time." It can be exhausting for those on the receiving end and finding themselves required to respond at any and all times. It can be wearing, exhausting, mind-numbing, and perhaps "soul-sucking." I also know people who will not have it any other way!

They want to be "on" all the time. They are driven, competitive, Type A, or Type AAA. They appear to be tremendous successes in their field. I know people at the top of their field whom I've repeatedly heard say things such as "I sleep every other night." We must consider the cost of such approaches to life and work. Some successes and the appearance of success can come at tremendous prices. Still, there are others who've successfully grabbed life by the horns and over time dug themselves out of this "conveyor belt" of always being on and in time "gotten their lives back."

I recently talked with a teacher as she reflected on the schedules middle schoolers and high schoolers maintain. She wondered how they do it all and is convinced these kids are being overtaxed and missing out on some things. And, most of them don't get enough sleep in a time of physical, psychological, and intellectual growth and development. Some families have made the good decision to be considerate about what their kids will be involved in and what they want, about what is doable and what is not. They have helped their kids to take the time and effort to consider their involvements and how they want to live.

Adults can deal with the same dynamics as they not only work their jobs, but also become involved in "jobs around their jobs"—jobs and involvements that "feed" their jobs, including industry organizations, amd civic and church involvements, to name a few. We find ourselves asking, "Where does it stop?" It's up to us to decide; if we don't, it never will.

Prepare for restorative sleep.

Excessive time spent in video games and screen time is negatively affecting sleep habits. We need to get from behind the screens well in advance of bedtime for best sleeping results. Likewise, we need to monitor our eating habits before going to bed.

Several years ago, I was having trouble with my voice. As a singer, that was really bugging me. Sometimes at 10 in the morning, I sounded like Joe Cocker on a bad day. I visited an ear-nose-and-throat (ENT) specialist who diagnosed me with a "silent reflux" problem. I told the doctor I wanted to correct the problem without long-term medication. I did take one round of the prescribed medicine, and my symptoms diminished, but I also did something more: I researched the silent reflux problem and learned that I had to quit eating further in advance of bedtime.

I hadn't regularly eaten supper late, but I had too often snacked till later than I should. Research pointed to not eating for three hours prior to bedtime, which for me meant no eating after 8 p.m. I followed that plan, and with rare exception, my voice has been clearer than in several years. It has also reduced sleeping difficulties and respiratory ailments. Research also indicates that we can prepare for enhanced sleep quality by reducing light and noise, maintaining comfortable temperatures, and keeping pets and TVs out of the bedroom

Invest in rest.

I tend to squeeze too much into a day and to stay up too late, but at 10:30 p.m. my reminder goes off to "invest in rest"—if I'm not already working my way there. We should see rest as an investment. I get it when people quip that you can sleep when you're dead. Well, facts seem to show that we'll live longer if we get proper rest now. Additionally, our quality of life will go up, and our freshness and creativity will increase. Our personalities are better when we're not tired and grumpy and cranky, thus our relationships are better.

Athletes emphasize again and again how important proper sleep and recovery are to them. We can only operate on sleep deprivation for so long. It's much better to keep sleep patterns steady and consistent as much as possible, going to bed and rising about the same time every day. Contrary to what many people think, we cannot sleep in on the weekend and make up for sleep deprivation during the week. Analyze how much sleep you're getting; most of us need more.

Thankfully, sleep usually comes easily for me, but I would recommend doing these things to get more and better sleep: During the day, find peace and quiet or pleasant moments. Then, before bedtime, change the pace of your day by winding down before bedtime.

I love pretty sunsets, preferably with my wife and others I love, on a bike path, over a pasture, over the mountains, along a seashore. I love to watch the birds around our home, especially as the sun sets. I've always cherished the big and little moments of beauty, of togetherness, of music, and more. Indeed, often and regularly, "my heart overflows." Relishing pleasant moments makes my head and heart satisfied and makes my restfulness and sleep more satisfying.

Then, there's that "good kind of tired" that we speak of after we've done manual labor or engaged in a form of exercise that left us rewarded physically. We do well by ourselves to let that kind of tiredness come often to enhance our sleep.

Clear your head before bedtime.

In my business dealings I tell my clients about my "So I Can Sleep at Night" policy. I will always tell them the things I know to be pitfalls or other problems I see. These are the kinds of things that many people in business keep quiet about in order to make that next sale. Meanwhile, they have to live with themselves, and their clients try to live with the consequences.

So that I can sleep at night, I must disclose concerns I see. But I also tell my clients it's up to them; they may choose not to listen to me. My policy is all about things that count. That commitment to honesty and doing my best helps me sleep well at night. I don't have to be ashamed of myself. I don't have to look over my shoulder and wonder if my clients ever found out that a problem I could have helped them avoid ended up costing them thousands of dollars. It's because I genuinely care about people, and so that I can live with myself and sleep at night.

Setting limits has also helped me prepare for better rest. I can still be flexible and adaptable and even gritty in my dealings, but at the same time maintain my self-respect. At times I've dismissed dysfunctional clients, which has enabled me to focus my energies and do more business, and best of all has reduced my stress and given me more peace. I've also gotten better about "diffusing the upsetting."

This is a variety of skills, centering around getting quickly to the heart of problems and applying good problem-solving techniques, being steady enough on my feet to help redirect or diffuse unnecessary anger, not taking ownership of others' drama and lack of character, and not letting negative "voices" run wild in my head. I don't allow these to be problems for me—so I can sleep at night.

Make time for exercise.

We all need exercise—and for the rest of our lives. It will make us thrive, adding to our energy instead of taking it away. The problem for many of us is that we've been exposed to ways of exercising that we find to be drudgery. We haven't discovered exercises that we can enjoy and do long term. We were made for exercise, not for the sedentary ways most of us have adopted. (Sitting is the new smoking. Strong is the new skinny.) Exercise is the most natural thing for us to do every day.

What was your introduction to exercise and working out? For many people, it came from playing sports. Some coaches help students discover lifetime exercises to enjoy throughout adulthood, but most are known only for what they make players do to prep for, say, football: eat big and go run. But what may have worked for someone in 1977 for football doesn't work at a different stage in life.

When you were trying to gain weight to get from 130 to 145 pounds, you needed to wolf down some steak. And, you ran to build endurance and spent time in the weight room. But this doesn't work in adulthood. I often see adults pounding the pavement and looking like it's not as fun anymore; they seem to be working out for football that they'll never play. And, some adults are still eating like they're 14 and starving, and trying to gain weight for football. Something needs to change.

Where we live, as I come rolling down the path on my bike, I meet men in their 30s, 40s, 50s out jogging, with a painful look on their face, still overweight and just pounding the heck out of their knees. It's not working! Now, I have friends who are runners who do it well. They're light on their feet and seem to have little trouble. But for many of us, running just doesn't work. So, look at the alternatives, and do one or more of them.

There's a lady in my neighborhood who I've observed for several years. I see her out simply walking. But so far, she's not been able to conquer being overweight. As she walks, she moves her head left to right as if disagreeing with something or saying "I've gotta walk, but I don't have to like it." Her facial expression, as well, tells me she's not having fun. I so wish I could help her enjoy it more—she's doing a great lifetime exercise by walking. If she could improve her diet and maybe also start walking in different places, to add interest, or walking with someone, to add in social benefit, she'd surely meet with success. Anyway, I hope she keeps doing it, and progresses. How about you? Let's get you going.

Make time for exercise—the time will pass anyway. If you think you're too busy to exercise, think again. It's your life! Care enough about yourself to take the time to exercise. And, in addition to many quality-of-life benefits, exercising will help reduce illness and make you stronger should you face illness. You'd be surprised what you can do in 15 minutes toward the exercise you need.

I'm going to walk you through what's been working for me for a long time in terms of both cardio exercises and workouts. If you don't copy me, then let this give you ideas on what you can and want to do. I would remind you, though, to consult your doctor before beginning an exercise program, especially if you've not been regularly exercising. Then, get to moving!

Rev up your engine with cardio exercise.

Let's work on your engine. Surely you know that doing cardio is good for your heart—and that "cardiac" is not good for your heart! Cardio exercises help your heart if done properly and under the right conditions. For starters, don't let Day 1 find you stepping out the door on a 100-degree day. But doing something for your heart is primary. You'll need to hydrate properly before, during, and after exercise whether it's aerobic or anaerobic. Move is the key word. If nothing else, just lace up your shoes and walk out the door, go somewhere, and come back. There is an array of choices to get good cardio.

Walking is tops for many people. Swimming is a favorite of my friend. Running delights some. Walking or running on a treadmill is the ticket for some. For inclement weather, I have an old stationary bike that I sometimes use. I call it the Hamsterbike because I like to throw off on it, because I do find it boring. But it's better than nothing, and that old Hamsterbike now has nearly 15,000 miles on it. Walking or running the stairs at a stadium or in a hotel or hospital or office building has great benefits. The list of ways to move and get cardio goes on and on.

Cardio exercise benefits your heart, your engine, first and foremost, but it also benefits your entire body and its functions—blood vessels, circulation, breathing, digestion, skin, and more. It makes you more vibrant and energetic and enduring at any age than you would be without it. Cardio is also a good sleep-inducer!

Benefit from cycling.

I love cycling! For more than 20 years I've ridden my bike three times most weeks. Cycling has become an integral, cherished part of my life. Even better, for more than seven years, my wife has usually joined me on those rides. In addition to what we'd call regular rides, we've ridden in some wonderful places further afield in Georgia, and in several surrounding states. We enjoy what we call "adventures."

From the time I got my first banana seat bike in the 60s, I loved my bike. It immediately became my "horse," on which I could explore our farm and the much larger adjacent ranch. I was delighted when I got to ride in my hometown's Youth Day Parade and cruise some streets I was used to seeing from the backseat of our Pontiac. What a feeling of freedom, even if under the parade guidelines. My bike set me free, especially since I'm terrible at running. It lets me go at as high a speed as I can muster and at times even faster than I really want to go. And I've ridden fast enough a few times to scare you. I'd have everybody out on bikes of some kind if it were up to me.

Cycling has changed my life. I've ridden much more in my adulthood than in my childhood and teenage years. Cycling has taken a guy who wasn't athletic into adulthood and offered me both fun and health care all at the same time. I've been able to ride much longer and further than I ever did growing up. Cycling has made me stronger in cardio, in my legs, and in character. I have been able to have endurance even in my 50s that I didn't have when I was 15, and I've gained muscle I never imagined. In addition, cycling has been a regular stress reducer.

A big benefit I've discovered in cycling is the great friendships I've developed over the years. Many of the best friends I know I've gained on a bike. Many of the best times I've had and the nicest people I've met came through cycling. If you're not just into heart rate and finish lines and personal best times, you can have some great conversations before, sometimes during, and after cycling. Riding with my wife has been the best cycling joy of all. We used to ride more often with our daughters during their growing-up years. And, I've had some memorable rides (and adventures) with the young men who are now our sons-in-law. I'm yearning for more of those with all of my family.

In addition to the friends I've gained through cycling, there are other benefits. Cycling adds a fun factor that I am certain walking or running simply cannot match. It makes the breezes blow through your hair. When you get to zoom, there can be excitement. Cycling enables you to cover much more ground than if you were on foot. Even when I've come home and said I had a bad day on the bike, it was still a better day than if I hadn't ridden.

There are also long-term health benefits from cycling. In addition to some of the mechanics we've covered already, I'll point out that countless times I've taken long-distance rides with people in their 60s and 70s—and they weren't creeping along. Cycling also burns calories, even in a 30-minute ride. Join me for two, three, or more hours on a ride, and that number can go way up. (Hills really are your friend!). Plus, cycling will give you muscles you cannot grow by walking.

Beer keg quads can happen, even if, like me, you don't drink beer. Mountain biking especially builds bone density, due to its HIIT (High Intensity Interval Training) nature. The rougher ride and the additional up-and-down off the seat are all factors in the additional bone-building benefits of mountain biking. Road cycling is not known to build bones, but still has quite a great list of benefits.

Earlier, I described my first biking experiences, mainly around our farm. Gravel roads and fields were home to me. The advent of mountain biking in the 80s was an immediate draw for me. A long-time subscriber to *Outside* magazine, I vividly remember a two-page ad back in the 80s from one of the top bike manufacturers that caught my imagination. A few more years and dozens of magazine articles about mountain biking inspired me. In the mid-90s I traded in my old road bike, first and briefly for a hybrid bike, then a mountain bike. I rode that bike for several years, then 10 years on the next mountain bike before I broke it (!), then another for about eight years. And, last year I got the mountain bike I'd dreamed of for 30 years. But oh, the experiences I've had mountain biking. I wish I could take more folks to some of the beautiful places I've pedaled. Though I have both a mountain bike and a road bike, I've often said if I could only have one, it'd be the mountain bike. But why choose?

I ride my mountain bike on the paths around our town and on rural gravel roads mostly south of our home. But it's the single-track trails in the mountains that are the most special. For example, on our 30th wedding anniversary trip, my wife and I stayed in Damascus, Virginia, along the famous

Virginia Creeper Trail. We rode east and west along that 34-mile idyllic rail trail twice each way over four days. We look forward to doing that again!

Road bikes offer an entirely different experience than mountain bikes. I love my pretty metallic blue road bike. I keep it waxed immaculately and love to see it gleam in the sun as I ride it. Road bikes are for paved roads mainly or smooth bike lanes. Due to where they work best, they require more alertness on rides, with the ever-present cars and their often distracted and incompetent drivers. In 15 years of road cycling, though, I've had very few scary moments. I ride very safely and alertly. I make myself very visible and position myself in the road for utmost safety. Still, it requires more focus and self-protection than mountain biking does.

The most enjoyable places on my road bike in our area include the Silver Comet rail trail, running west from the west side of Atlanta, and various country road routes. For years I've enjoyed road biking with a great friend of mine, plus two or three other friends at times. Also, I've done many larger organized rides around the area, including charity fundraisers. Since my wife now also has a road bike, we've enjoyed riding in various places—we've been known to knock out a 35-mile loop in rapid fashion on a Sunday afternoon. We've enjoyed riding bikes in other places too—paths, gravel roads, and wherever.

Having lived in Peachtree City, Georgia since 1995 with its signature path system—now totaling more than 100 miles—cycling has been an essential part of our lifestyle. I've been involved in getting bike lanes added to a few parts of our city and in the efforts that helped us achieve official "Bike Friendly City" designation. I've also been involved in championing neighboring Newnan, Georgia's effort at a path system, called the Linc, which will total more than 25 miles of paths when completed. Now, if we could just interconnect all our cities with paths, what a different and better world we could have!

Gravel roads are also favorite riding places. The wave called "gravel grinding" has begun to catch up with what I've been doing since childhood. For example, my wife and I love to gravel-road ride in a couple counties below us to Georgia's longest covered bridge. Such fun! There are many places to ride a bike. Get on your bike and ride!

Let me give a few brief notes about "bike paraphernalia" and your bike. First, don't order online, but find the nearest good bike shop and buy from a human who will offer you a good product and properly fit and adjust it. While there, purchase bike shorts, tights/pants, bike bottles, and lights (if you ride at night). Shirts are debatable: I tend to like athletic, breathable ones, due to my build. For winter riding, gloves and jackets and layering will save your life! Go visit your local bike shop.

Walk for fitness and fun.

Many people have said that for fitness, there's nothing better than walking. All you need are comfortable shoes and clothes. Just open the door and go. Walking is something all ages can do. It's one of the most convenient and available exercises. Make it enjoyable and you'll be more prone to do it regularly. It's something that, hopefully, you can do the rest of your life. I suggest walking with friends or family for good conversation and motivation. Then there's hiking.

Our family has enjoyed many hikes over the past 30-plus years. When our daughters were born, we hiked and carried them to waterfalls and other beautiful places before they could even walk. When our first grandchild was born, our daughter said, "Dad, you know we'll have to take her to a waterfall soon." And now the other daughter is saying the same thing about our second grandchild. We've enjoyed hikes all over Georgia and in several other states.

When we first started hiking, we found out about places through books and magazines. We took hiking books with us or ripped out pages from magazines so we could know where to go. Now, directions for hikes are right there in our phone. We've had wonderful adventures and made great memories. Since we've never done overnight or multi-day hikes, we've always traveled lightly— no big backpack required, just water and snacks. (We've seen only a handful of snakes and one bear in 30 years. Don't worry. Just use commonsense.)

Other special moments have occurred when we have taken folks out for their first hike ever—children, teens, even some north of 60. I was tickled to get them out there. With a little research and forethought, you can find hikes with distances and terrain that fit your ability, time, and desire. The next adventure, the next beautiful spot around the next bend in the trail will give you motivation.

Again, comfortable walking/hiking shoes and clothes and appropriate-for-distance water and snacks are all you need. I've even seen some short hikes that were handicapped accessible—a wonderful thing. Our family joke about hikes is that, if we see more than five people on the trail, it's too crowded. We like to get far out—nothing touristy for us. So, walk around town, walk in new places, walk on vacation, take some hikes.

Walking and hiking burn fat as good as anything. Just after we were married, due to accessibility, my wife and I did a lot of walking. For a brief time, I got skinny! I was 21, 6′ 2″ and just over 160 pounds. Subsequent working out and cycling have added a number of pounds on the ole boy, but yes, consistent walks will burn calories.

I hope you live somewhere with pretty places to go walking. If not right where you live, maybe there are parks or other places nearby that will delight your senses as you walk. This adds to your enjoyment and relaxation and motivates you to go again and again. When we walk, and when we ride, I like to mix it up and go somewhere different every time. I'm certain that has helped keep it fresh all these years.

Walkability matters. Interest in walkability is spreading. According to recent reports, as much as 60 percent of all new construction in metro Atlanta is now happening in walkable places. Additionally, miles of multi-use trails are being planned across a span of metro Atlanta. And, of course I continue to cheer on the expansion of rail trails and the like in Georgia and across our nation. Walkability is a great word. Fall in love with it.

Incorporate workouts into your exercise routine.

We've talked a lot about cardio, about exercises that help our heart, our engine. But we need to work out, too. We need to get strong. Let's look at working out, so you can incorporate it into your daily routine.

Skinny, fat, skinny fat: I've been all three. I've been a lanky little boy, I've been a "junk food junky," I've been briefly skinny in early adulthood, and I've been overweight at various times before and since. I don't mean dramatic gains and losses of weight or the old "roller coaster" gain-and-lose thing some folks do. But I have had my ups and downs over the years, with maybe my best success in my 50s!

Working out is key to success in long-term fitness. After back spasms in my 30s, I began exercises that strengthened my core and back. Without becoming an Olympic lifter, I discovered that I could add a certain helpful amount of strength without becoming overly bulky and all the maintenance that goes with that. You probably need to be stronger, too. We all need "maintenance strength work." Again, it's what we were made for.

I would organize strength maintenance around four areas: arms, core, hips, and legs. To gain flexibility, you may want to weave in yoga moves or Pilates workouts or fascia stretching on a foam roller or even on a big Swiss exercise ball—there are many options. Basic strength maintenance will give you some "buff," make daily chores and lifting easier, and preserve muscles, joints, and bones as you age.

In a bit, I'll share with you my favorites for building and maintaining strength. But first, think about people you've seen in old pictures. They were slimmer because they engaged in manual labor such as farming. The way they eked out an existence required them to move, walk, lift objects, and push and pull on things. That's what we're designed to do. But in the last few decades, the 1970s and beyond, some of us started going to pot! So, we need to replace some of the old manual labor with working out, lifting weights, pushing sleds, sledgehammering tires, whatever it may be. Working out can counter some of the effects of sitting—"the new smoking."

We sit so much! We sit when we drive, we sit when we work, we sit when we're off work. The latest medical reports confirm that sitting is killing us. We must overcome gravity. Look for opportunities to get up, to walk around, to move. Prescribe for yourself more movement in your "off hours." It's so easy and habit-forming to go to work, fight your way through the commute back home, and then vegetate in front of the TV and the iPad. Instead, grab some movement to overcome a day's worth of "downward forces."

Some people work out at a gym or CrossFit "box." Others improvise workouts in parks such as on park benches or by climbing stadium stairs and such. Some of us work out at home. Where's your gym? You don't have one? Get a workout place of your own, and fast. Where should it be? It's the one that works for you and that is readily accessible.

When people ask me, I tell them I work out at Jim's Gym. Maybe you need the buzz of people or the assistance and motivation of trainers at a gym. Maybe the camaraderie and constant variations at a CrossFit box help you. Some people like the peace and quiet and scenery and the improvisation that a workout in a park or other place affords. Wherever your gym may be, just be consistent with your workouts. Although I usually work out at home,

I've done it in hotel rooms, and my wife and I enjoy running the steps wherever we visit. I've done workouts in all sorts of places because that's what I have to do to be consistent. So, what are my workouts like? Here are some favorites:

- I start my workout with squats. These are helpful, go-to, foundational exercises. Air squats are done without holding additional weight. For weighted squats, I use a Wreckbag, kettlebells, and dumbbells, and now I enjoy squats with a slamball.

- Most days I do 50 oblique twists. These have been helpful in core toning and strengthening. I always recommend doing them in a controlled fashion to avoid over-rotating and hurting your back.

- Over the last few years, burpees have become a favorite part of my workout routine. To do burpees, basically, throw yourself down on the floor, jump back up again, and keep doing this until . . . Burpees are a great full body exercise. How about doing 20? You may do more, or less, but do them if you can.

- Pushups are good. As with burpees, there are variations you can do if currently the purist version is too tough. Work your way up to 20 or more.

- Donkey kicks offer the lower half of the burpees move without the upper body part. Get in a push-up position, kick back with both feet, repeatedly, maybe 25 times. This will work your midsection and get your heart beating. These together with pushups help prepare you for burpees if you're just getting started or starting back.

- Hollow rocks involve lying on your back, holding up your arms and legs simultaneously, and rocking to work the core. A good number would be 30.

- I love my kettle bells. I've got a couple in different weights that I alternate between. I've also got a couple of medicine balls in different sizes and weights, and using these old but now very popular tools—perhaps a set of 20—provides a good workout.

• The steps in your home can be a great place to work out or throw in a different exercise or two for variation. Try crawling on all fours upstairs (called bear crawls) or crawling downstairs. Or, sit on the bottom-third stair and do about 30 leg raises or reverse crunches.

• From sturdy couch backs or chair backs, I've often done dips. Be careful here to control the dip to avoid damaging your shoulders.

Working out always makes me glad. Some days are better than others, but it's always better when I do. Being consistent is also very rewarding. You'll be surprised how much working out you can do in just 15 minutes, and of course longer can be even more rewarding. The feel of vibrancy after daily workouts can be nirvana. Do variations of my workout or make up your own routine. Variety is a good thing. Just make sure it challenges you some, gets your heart rate up, gets you breathing hard, and maybe even makes you sweat. All of these will benefit you and make you happy you did them. Don't expect results immediately, but keep doing them for the rest of your life.

Exercise to boost self-esteem and improve health.

Being fit will take you higher, elevate your experiences, and add crispness and vitality to your days. Being fit frees you to feel better, move better, and be more confident than you otherwise would be. Being fit just adds another dimension to living than most folks ever know. It's truly how you and I were meant to be. Embrace it, desire it, achieve it, enjoy it. And, share it. It's why I've enjoyed taking folks on bike rides and hikes over the years. It's why I've often shared bits and pieces of what I've learned in my fitness journey. Maybe it's time you experienced what I'm talking about here.

It doesn't take forever to be strong: the time passes either way. So, wherever you are today, or whatever you're doing, the clock is ticking. Life happens. Take care of yourself: the time passes either way, so get through it in the best condition possible. It'll make your life richer and happier. It could happen for you, if you'll make the effort.

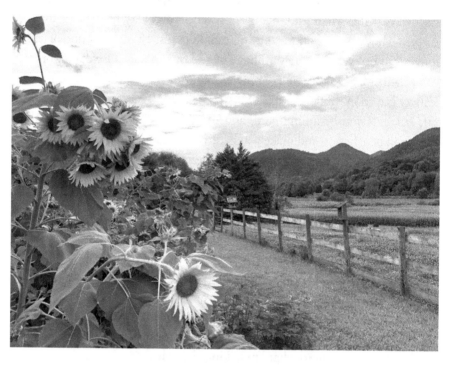

Foster a healthy mind, spirit, and emotions.
Feed your thoughts and focus as you take care of yourself.

Chapter 2

Take Care of Your Mind, Spirit, and Emotions

I meet so many unhappy people. I've learned that I cannot make them happy, but I always wish I could share a little happiness with them. Some of them seem to have drifted and warped from whatever tender, innocent children they were once. Some are caught up in playing a persona, living out a controlled personality they believe is essential to their career or for whom they are trying to keep impressed. I have to wonder what happened to them.

Recently I mused to a friend from high school, "When did so many of our fellow students turn into Archie Bunker?" When Archie Bunker wasn't a re-run on TV, very few of our classmates would have shared his attitudes. Now, due to experiences, bitterness, peer pressure, cable news, and other influences, many of them sound like Archie Bunker.

Are we happy being like this? I don't believe so. Thankfully, I also know and deal with many happy, equitable, loving people. I know who I want to be like.

While you're taking care of yourself, take care of your mind, spirit, and emotions. Doing so will change your relationships, your feelings, your perspective, your business dealings, and your life. It can affect your happiness, yes, but also your emotional intelligence, your stress and optimism levels, your perseverance, your health, your spirituality, and more. Taking care of your mind, spirit, and emotions will help you be a more authentic person, more like you were meant to be, maybe even "untamed," not so calculating, not so stiff—even freer and happier. Let's look at some things that will help us take care of our mind, spirit, and emotions.

Enable children to be happy.

I love children. My wife and I raised two wonderful daughters, so we think and so people tell us. In the past two years we welcomed our first grandchildren. We know we'll shower them with love, too. Unfortunately, far too many children have happiness robbed from them, usually by adults.

For years I've heard people share the difficult emotional burdens adults dumped on them as children. I once witnessed a dad tell his son, "I wish you'd never been born." I'll never forget it. I can only hope that father and son later reconciled, but odds are they didn't. Once some things come out of the mouth, like toothpaste out of the tube, you can't put it back in.

I don't believe we should pressure little children to be geniuses or super athletes by the time they're six. I've seen too many children who were abused physically, verbally, emotionally. I've seen what happens to them as they reach adulthood and beyond. Life is hard enough without all that.

So, those of us who have children should strive every day to build them up, give them a foundation for healthy personalities, and teach them lots of life lessons along the way. Our time with our children is precious, and they grow up quickly. Are we adding pluses to their columns, or minuses? Are we building them up or tearing them down?

A fellow college student was a sad case. He was a very intelligent fellow, but I quickly began to learn why he was so socially awkward and often volatile. I heard story after story about how his dad had verbally abused him. Another longtime friend revealed to me in recent years the physical abuse he'd received as a child from his dad. He's had so much to overcome, but is one of the finest people I've ever known. Two young men I first knew as teenagers also come to mind. I've quipped more than once to my wife that "if I had his mom," I wouldn't have turned out as well.

Thankfully, I've also known people who have overcome their upbringing and healed and thrived, in spite of the emotional and physical beatings from significant adults. It can be done, but it can be so hard.

Seek help to overcome negative experiences.

Beyond abuses and bad childhood experiences, many things can add up over time to put downward pressures on our emotions and outlook in life— excruciating times; experiences that make you want to run away, ball up in the corner, scream, cry, throw things, and more. I know people who've had failed marriages, failed businesses, and tragedies who often display the bitterness and hopelessness that go along with such difficulties. It's not hard to see why their perspectives and outlooks are so negative, bitter, and angry. But these mindsets don't serve us well. Aside from any dynamics we need to consider and work through when it comes to overcoming and healing, we have to realize that we are only compounding problems by becoming bitter, angry, sarcastic, or depressed.

It's okay to be happy! Failure to be happy is a symptom. Oddly enough, there have been a couple times in my life when someone around me griped that I was too happy. They weren't complaining that I was too loud or talkative, just too happy. I've had a couple times when, after muddling and struggling through some ongoing difficult situations, I decided to make a change. In overcoming dysfunction and toxic situations, a couple of people questioned if the reason for my decision was depression. Not for a minute!

Not every day in our lives is rosy, but in it all, through it all, above it all, beyond it all, we can find and know happiness. Being unhappy day in and day out should be a sign that something is wrong, something is out of line, something is not okay.

So, if you're unhappy consistently, do some self-examination and introspection. But also talk with a few select, stable, trustworthy friends. And, seek professional help if needed to identify, sort out, analyze, and work through the factors that are making you consistently unhappy. Too many lives are either lived out in long-term misery or ended unnecessarily and tragically in suicide.

My mind flashes immediately now to people I've known who I wish could have lived out their lives happily and didn't. Additionally, I remember twice when I was the second or third person at the scene of a suicide, and I remember the tragedy for all involved. You deserve to find happiness, and it's OK to get the help you need.

Happiness can be possible in the midst of struggle. Several times in my life I've found myself in the middle of toxic, dysfunctional environments and situations. I learned the value of fortitude, perseverance, self-awareness, anger management, perspective, patience, assertiveness, when to speak and when not to speak, and more. I learned how to plod along. I learned to focus on those people and things in my life that mattered most.

When I look back on those times, I also see the happiness I enjoyed in the midst of it all. I appreciate folks who've thanked me for "steadying the boat." I relish the moments with people from those times and the timeless relationships we've maintained. I realize that one of the victories from difficult situations has been that I didn't let the difficulties become all-consuming. I kept stirring in other ingredients, including love, forgiveness, laughter, encouragement, and clarity, plus a few moments of assertive force at exactly the right time. I learned to be happy "in spite of."

How about you? Is something or someone stealing your happiness? Are you letting them rob you? What can you do that is positive, helpful, healthy, and productive?

Unhappiness, anger, drama, and bitterness are seemingly epidemic in our society. Just spend a little time on social media, and I'm sure you'll see vitriol from some of your "friends" about politics or social issues or relationships or "who they don't like." Could that be you? Can you engage in civil, collected discussions about issues, or must you be an angry (name your demographic)?

I'm often amazed at social gatherings how often and how quickly someone brings up a zinger about some political or social hot-button issue. They're boiling just under the surface about it, and up it comes. Others reveal how they never can be satisfied, always complaining, always unhappy. Then there are those I walk away from repeatedly, noting under my breath "drama, drama, drama." Others are "cooking in their own juices" of bitterness about whatever.

Many times when I've reflected with my daughters about such folks, I've observed how it's a slow, painful death—a rough way to live. Yet, I insist there's still hope for any of us who want to heal and change our ways. It may take something drastic on our part and may take some time to develop new emotional habits, but it'll be worth the effort.

Foster healthy emotions.

We talk a lot about health, but it's usually about physical health: we don't tend to talk much about emotional health. Some tragic recent suicides by celebrities have brought out discussions about people needing to get help. Just turn on the news and you'll witness reports of shootings, road rage incidents, domestic disputes, toxic work environments and scandals, egomaniacs in high places—all evidence of unhealthy emotions running rampant.

Most of us agree that if we eat junk food all the time, our bodies won't be healthy—though that still may not stop us. Most of us would also agree that eating genuinely healthy foods will increase our health and fitness. Yet we fail to realize that what we feast on mentally affects our emotions. I know of people who watch hour after hour and day after day certain news channels and talk radio programs that feed their fears and anger and determine what is reality to them.

I've seen people go from being generous and free-breathing to becoming angry, bitter, calculating people. Yes, people can change—positively and negatively. I regret every time I see someone who has much good about them but they get hoodwinked, hoodooed, and hijacked by the forces of anger and bitterness. We must be constantly vigilant to foster healthy emotions in our hearts and lives. Don't let emotions tame you: keep the wildness!

I remember back in the 60s when my folks had our driveway paved. My grand uncle owned a paving company. I had a little "racetrack" that I'd worn out with my tricycle and wagon and pedal car. It stretched from our patio, past the carport, out to and around a small magnolia tree, and then out to our vegetable garden. I began "negotiating" for it to be paved, too. Much to my surprise then and now, it got paved! I think my grand uncle was mainly responsible for siding with me. The crew shoveled out small amounts of asphalt along my little track and then used a small roller to smooth it out and pack it down. I remember the puzzlement of more than one man as my dad explained it all. No, it really didn't make sense. But it was fun to this little boy!

My racetrack was different things to me on different days. Some days it was an interstate highway, still a relatively new feature on the American landscape at that time. My dad loved the interstates, because he loved speed. I picked up on that, too. Some days my racetrack was where I came bursting out of the Batcave (our patio) on my Fire Chief pedal car (Batmobile), as I was Batman rushing off to see Commissioner Gordon about the latest fiend posing a threat.

With the years we mature, and imaginary places and characters get replaced with earning a living and real-world concerns. We become serious adults with serious notions and furrowed brows. We obviously need to be become professional, insightful, hardworking, contributing, dependable people. Every day brings serious things to do at our businesses, civic involvements, church involvements, and more. But often there is a price we pay for all this maturity and seriousness and responsibility. Something happens to many of us. We become wooden, static, hollow, stiff, calculating, and worse. We become what I sometimes quip as "too damn serious." (I've abbreviated that syndrome as TDS. Perhaps I should be credited in psychology journals for coining the term.) Lest someone be horrified that I've used one expletive, let me get more technical and term it "too damned serious" because seriousness at the level some of us can take it to is indeed damning. It knows no grace, no relief, no humor. It's a touch ride. It's awfully somber.

Have you become that way in adulthood? Has the life been sucked out of you? Does it take too much to thrill you? Or to light up your smile? Would you never be caught dead riding a grocery cart across the parking lot?

A real estate agent once told me she never wears jeans to the grocery store, because she anticipates she'll run into clients and prospective clients. I run into them there, too, but sometimes I'm dressed for the office and sometimes I'm in shorts and a tee-shirt. Can we be comfortable in our own skin? How far must we go in the sometimes all-consuming effort to "dress for success"?

Our kids watch us as they grow up and, though they may not be able to put their finger on it or give an analysis, they see how we change with age: not only our bodies but also our personalities grow heavier with time. Too often the flash goes out of our eyes, the spark leaves our personalities, the hope leaves our hearts, and tenderness gets taken away. Another way to put it is "the wild gets taken out of us." Who we were meant to be and who we really are gets covered up and replaced with something we think we're supposed to be in order to fit in and succeed, and it never really fits right.

It doesn't have to be this way. We can be our best real self. We can have a twinkle in our eyes. We can be lighter on our feet. There's a balance to adulthood that we can maintain, if we're vigilant and thoughtful. I've fought what could be soul-sucking in business by trying to be myself, feeding my soul and my brain, having multiple interests, enjoying outdoor activities and adventures, working at physical fitness, engaging in business practices that agree with my soul, demanding integrity from myself and others, and maintaining family, church, and civic involvements regularly. A lot of regular introspection has helped with that.

When asked to do certain things, I ponder how and who I want to be and determine whether the opportunities fit or not. Maybe there are sacrifices or sometimes "losses" I've taken, but I've always gained in important ways. And that stuff about not letting them tame you, about not losing the "wildness"—it's both important and possible. It's about not being caged up or being "over-domesticated" or losing something we're born with. We can still be our genuine, vibrant, and clear-eyed selves.

Live in a state of thankfulness.

Former President Jimmy Carter was asked at age 93 to share what prayer is like for him now. He said in the past it was much more about asking, but now it is mostly about giving thanks and being aware of the goodness of God. I couldn't agree more. I discovered long ago to "relish" and be thankful every day. This is key in my faith tradition, and something practiced by the people who've impressed me most. Our perspective, our attitude, so much about us changes and grows when we develop this kind of thankfulness.

Savoring good things that happen, good things that are said and done, people who are dearest to us, moments when we move beyond ourselves to help others (or when someone helps us), moments when we gain a larger vision or wisdom that takes us beyond where we were before: these and many more deserve to be relished, cherished, absorbed, dwelled upon, and not forgotten. One good experience after another, each insight will build upon another. Our perspective and outlook will grow exponentially

I relish moments of goodness and charity when people in need are genuinely helped, not just given a handout. I relish moments with family and friends and others. I relish moments of "adventure" in natural beauty—waterfalls have long been favorite spots I've frequented, among others.

Music is also huge in my life, as I've been singing since I was 12. Other cherished moments come from my cycling experiences alone. I've learned first to be present and in tune in the middle of moments, and I've learned to ponder and treasure moments after they've happened. It can be the big things, but it also can be the little things—the little moments that we should not dare miss their value. More than once someone has quipped to me, "Jim, it doesn't take much for you." I've considered that a tremendous compliment. This means it doesn't take much to make me happy, to light me up, to make my day.

If you'll learn this secret, life will become richer for you. You won't need as much. At some point you'll find your "heart overflows." You'll become thankful and not so demanding. You'll realize how much you have and be less needy. Thankfulness will revolve less around things received and more around moments and exchanges that happen. In the midst of the most materialistic and dissatisfied society in history, you'll find yourself with an entirely different and contrasting outlook. And, you'll be in a better position to offer more of what that very society desperately needs.

Deal with anger appropriately.

We see so much of it. More than any time I can remember, it seems people are out-of-control angry. Tragic shootings, incidents of road rage, disturbances on airplanes, acts of domestic violence, and many other terrible things happen every day. Look a little further, and you'll see signs of anger on a quieter, seething level.

Things people believe, prejudices that divide, the way voting decisions are made, the way managers deal with employees, the gradual breakup of marriages: these are too often fueled by anger. It seems that everywhere you look, in every arena of life, somebody is at a low boil about something. Experiencing healthy anger about things that are wrong and need to be righted is different from harmful anger that is hurting you or other people. That is the challenge we must grapple with.

I've had my moments. People often comment that I'm a person who keeps his cool, keeps the boat steady, laughs a lot. I think it's true, and I'm happy with those reviews. But yes, I've had my moments, and I've needed to learn from them.

I recall an incident early in my marriage when a neighbor was "mooching" off me, taking advantage of me repeatedly for favors. It became ridiculous at how he just assumed it could go on forever. I forget how it resolved, but it did. But what I remember more vividly was my own internal discussion over how angry and resentful I'd become. I lectured myself to "don't do that again!"

I've had other situations that took more time and patience and fortitude. I've known times when I was at least briefly so angry I could spit. If I told you about them, I think you'd get angry just hearing the stories. I've had my share of angering situations, but I've also realized that I had to move on. I had to resolve my anger healthfully.

Unresolved, corrosive anger messes up everything. It consumes our thoughts, changes our attitudes, affects our speech, and boils our blood. Acidic, even explosive anger ruins relationships and creates job turnovers, confusion, anxiety, depression, and more. Hateful anger makes people gather and connive and plot and devise all sorts of corrupt schemes that can affect a few or even thousands. It's gone on throughout history.

How much is anger affecting your own history? Is anger what you want to determine the course of your life?

Dig into any misdeed you choose—any evil, conniving scheme—in relationships, organizations, business, politics, or world history, and you'll see anger fueling it. Anger makes people feel they need more than they have, makes them feel somebody's taking something from them, and leads to plots to take over, expel, beat down, or whatever it takes. Anger distorts our vision and clouds our worldview.

Has anger got you in its gnarly clutches? Look deep. Wherever you see anger, decide to turn toward hope and healing and a brighter day.

Avoid building a life around anger.

We don't set out to do it. We all start out as innocent little kids. Then, it happens: we experience different influences that shape our young lives. Maybe it's in adulthood before we experience troubling forces. It could be tragedies, job difficulties or loss, relationship breakups, societal changes, becoming a victim of a crime—many different things. But we can change positively or negatively. We can bloom or fail.

Sometimes we stumble into anger and bitterness, and it grows. We feed it by seeking out influences and people who reinforce our feelings. Our anger and bitterness take on a life of their own, and we become somebody perhaps very different from how we started out. Angry, bitter people usually won't admit it, but they've changed. They've become that way in response to whatever has happened or that they think has happened. They base too many decisions on anger.

Anger is no way to build a life. Make that a warning to yourself as you encounter it every day. There are so many other outcomes that can work better. Examine yourself, and get ahead of corrosive anger that may be robbing you.

Have you ever said, "No, I'm gonna cool down before I make that call"? That's good. But perhaps you've been the recipient of someone's misplaced or mishandled anger. So, there's anger we have to overcome and there's anger we have to handle in a healthy way.

Knee-jerk reactions are often fueled by anger. A man kicks his dog because it does something he doesn't like. A parent acts out violently at a child, all because of pent-up frustration and the inability to cope. The child is a helpless victim of physical and emotional trauma that is never forgotten. A group of parents make the news again because they got in a fight at their kids' baseball game. We look at the scene with disgust. Maybe we reflect on times when we didn't fight, but we got too angry about something at the kids' game. We must become aware of how we are reacting and feeling, and deal more productively and healthfully with our negative emotions.

Inward anger is a slow, nasty death. It includes seething anger just under the surface that seems to always be on a low boil. Anger inward is also what appears as depression. I call it anger we just choke down, and it gives us "psychological indigestion." This anger and the issues or dissatisfaction that fuel it never get "digested." As it worsens, inward anger ruins our health, and at its worst can lead to deep sadness and even suicide. Outward anger is more visible and evident. We see it in angry outbursts, hostile personalities, "throwing a fit," acts of rage and violence, and more.

Some people have both inward and outer anger. They're like volcanoes, perhaps cooking and building up pressure under the surface for years before they erupt. Does any of this describe you?

Get ahead of anger before it gets ahead of you. Deal with issues and feelings in ways that bring resolution. Don't just seethe and feast upon and multiply your anger. Identify it and then discuss it with the stated intent of resolving the anger and its causes. It does us no good to just complain and rehash and act unhappy and be "dramatic" and keep everybody around us unhappy.

I'm convinced that unresolved anger—inward or outward or both—is a slow and painful death. Could it be killing you and you don't recognize it? It could be that others around you see it and you don't. Decide to heal. Get help if you need it. Swallow some foolish pride, and start moving toward getting happy before it's too late.

Direct anger in healthy ways.

There are a multitude of secrets for managing anger in healthy, helpful, positive ways—possibly as many as there are things that make us angry. Over time I've learned to not let things anger me as easily. One crisis in particular taught me that some things matter and some things don't—and yes, the wisdom is to know the difference.

So, somebody pulled out in front of you in traffic. Your spouse said something that sets you off for the 10,000th time. You got up on the right side of the bed this morning, then stubbed your toe going around to the wrong side of the bed. Are you now mad and in a bad mood?

That mood thing: I've heard all my life folks announce about themselves, "I'm in a bad mood today." Then they go on to describe to others why they're in a bad mood and why everyone had better watch out. I used to work in a place where I would receive "memos" in advance that the boss was in a bad mood, which was a frequent occurrence. I would respond, "And?" Of course, I made note of that and prepared to respond to and work the boss with my own eventually successful strategy! But many times, I've discussed with people my own stance that I don't do moods and I don't expect others to have to put up with a mood from me.

I've never wanted it said about me: "Watch out for Jim; he's in a bad mood." I've long believed that, first, we should seek to live lovingly and kindly with each other as a basic rule of life. Then, whether big or small, if there are "issues" between us, we need to deal with them. Let's keep the negative emotions and drama out of it. Let's be constructive. And, don't let bad feelings stack up and "fester." Whether it's snarky passive-aggressive behavior or the inability to negotiate or just general irritability, let's move past those bad habits and deal with things in ways that bring healing and health and happiness to our interactions.

I remember an angry moment from my childhood. We were visiting with family, and I was playing out in the backyard. I discovered that meanwhile out front my dad and others had gone somewhere in the car, leaving me behind. Feeling I should have been included, somewhat angry, and maybe wanting to get some attention about it, I grabbed a pebble and threw it back at the ground as hard as I could. Thinking that would make an impression, I had no idea what would happen next. The pebble bounced up and hit my dear aunt in the head. She "ouched" but was otherwise uninjured. My mother immediately fussed at me. But I was already so ashamed of what I'd done. I learned much from that moment.

There are things we sometimes get angry about that are really not worth the stress. We need to learn to choose what we'll be angry about and how much. We can learn to control and channel our anger healthfully; to express our anger in the best ways in the moment and in the situation. "Flying off the handle" is rarely the best thing. We should always avoid any violence or words that will harm another. Expressing anger honestly and dealing with the issues involved is much better. And, we should never say anger is always bad. There are violations of truth and decency and kindness that should anger us and move us to action, individually, organizationally, and as a nation. We just have to channel anger in constructive and thoughtful ways. It can be a challenge, but life demands that we try to master it.

Avoid a diet of sarcasm.

Some of the first encounters with sarcasm I remember were at my dad's store. Starting work there at 10 years old gave me a sudden introduction to a myriad of personalities at a young age. It gave me good preparation and education about dealing with people of every shape and size and personality and demographic. There were lots of nice people, but others as well—and, yes, among them, the sarcastic.

At the time I didn't know the term sarcastic. I'm certain many of the sarcastic adults I encountered regularly also didn't think of the term sarcasm and didn't recognize it in themselves. But at some point, I began to recognize it as such and began to know its sour taste. I got a daily dose of sarcasm about economic ups and downs, the weather, the latest cars to hit the market, music, newcomers to the area, and a host of other things. Over cups of coffee and bottles of Coke, I heard thousands of reviews of everything under the sun through those years working at Greenway Grocery. Some customers even took it to another level that I'd call "pontificating."

At a young age I had to begin to filter and decipher and discern from all those things I heard every day. I learned to at least question within myself and evaluate all that stuff. By no means did I ever want to be someone who was naïve and just believed everything. But I also quickly realized I didn't want to turn sour at too young an age. I listened to those most sour individuals, who we could always count on to walk in and tell us the latest of what was wrong with everything—the Eeyore perspective. As they dwelt on the sarcastic side of things, I came to see what gave them that outlook. Various experiences in life soured them and made them not expect much.

Sarcasm can be briefly funny: we find it in satire, literature, and cartoons. In English lit studies I learned about satire. I've read editorial cartoons my whole life. Their satire, tinged at least with sarcasm, can make a point. I've studied how satire, over the centuries, has "spoken truth to power." There is a place for the nip, the sting, the bite of such observations. But you can't stay there; you can't make it a constant diet. There must be other ingredients in the mix.

Sarcasm is akin to, even fueled by, anger—it's sour. Sarcasm doesn't "believe all things and hope all things." In fact, sarcasm disbelieves. Sarcasm doubts, looks askance, bets it'll never happen. Sarcasm has seen things that give it just enough gripe and at least low-level anger that it keeps on looking for the worst in all but the things it loves. Is this you or someone you know?

Sarcasm lowers our esteem of ourselves and others. I'm not talking about the occasional snarky dig or wry humor. I love self-deprecating humor, as long as it's not growing negativity about myself; it's the same with humor aimed at others. Sarcasm works in a "minor key," reflecting and expecting less than our best.

For years I've heard people be sarcastic about their homes, their cars, their dogs, their cats (that's understandable), their clothes, their appearance, their teenagers, their spouses, and more. There's a tinge of sadness, the feeling that things could be happier and better. There's a weariness there. It could be reflective of the need to spruce up, clean out the garbage, open the windows, let's the sunshine in, maybe deal with some issues, and create some good memories together.

Spend some time listening to folks and yourself more closely. Listen to the drift of what's said. Could it move from a minor key to a major key? (For non-musicians, that's from a sad sound to a happier sound.).

Sarcasm fuels negativity, prejudice, societal patterns, and decisions. Whether it was at my dad's store or in thousands of conversations since or over lunch with a friend or in a meeting with a client or at a community or family gathering, I've always noted the sarcasm that seems to inevitably come up, usually completely unsolicited. It's like some folks have to go there, have to drift toward the ditch, just have to bring it up. Many times, I think people go there just to fit in; it gives them something to talk about. But cumulatively, the sarcasm adds up.

If we reflect on other groups, our coworkers, our neighbors, our kids sarcastically—call it negative energy or just negativity—it has an effect; it communicates; it influences. If we worked positively and constructively and thoughtfully in all these realms of life, they'd all be stronger. We need to contribute instead of tear down. Our families, workplaces, churches, communities, and even our state and nation would be better because of it.

Own your selfhood.

So, what do you want to be when you grow up? Many of us heard that question when we were young. (Maybe we are still growing up, and still answering that question.) Some of us knew early on what we wanted to be, and we've done exactly that. Others of us have grown up and done nothing like what we talked about when we were young. For others, it has been a winding road, maybe even full of adventure. We have to answer the question, "What do you want to be?" so we can at least have gainful employment. While we're answering "what," we also need to answer "who" we want to be in life.

(Yes, I want my daughters to be successful in their careers. As much or more, though, I want my daughters to be happy and fulfilled and to be people of character. I'm glad to report that's exactly who they are!)

Selfhood can be a struggle. Since I was a boy in the mid-60s, the misfit elf character in the old classic film, *Rudolph the Red Nosed Reindeer*, always intrigued me. He didn't want to be an elf; he wanted to be a dentist. Through ridicule and difficulty, that's exactly what he became.

I've seen many people through the years be a square peg in a round hole. I've seen people struggle with "what Daddy wanted me to do." Even more, in our rapidly changing times, I've seen people lose careers due to changing technology and markets. It can be hard to adapt; some do it better than others. There can be great successes and tremendous tragedies. In the midst of it all, there's also the challenge of being yourself—your real, genuine self.

Another character from a film classic comes to mind. In Disney's *The Lion King*, both Rafiki and Mufasa tell Simba to "remember who you are." I've referred to this scene through the years in conversations with my daughters and others. Of course, my girls have always laughed when I feebly attempted with my tenor voice to say "remember who you are" like James Earl Jones did. (I came much closer with my renditions of Rafiki by Robert Guillaume.).

Career choices and strategies and changes aside, I've always been clear that who I am and what I do are two different things. Maybe you're clear about that, too, but many people aren't, and it becomes problematic. I've had at least one career in which many of the people in that vocation cannot separate who they are from what they do. When they come home at night, many of them mentally and emotionally never leave work. It consumes their lives. If circumstances require them at some time to make a career change, or when they retire, I'm afraid they'll be lost, adrift, not knowing quite what to do. This proves unhealthy at any stage of life.

Who we are and what we do certainly feed each other, but they should not be one and the same. The average college graduates of today not only will have job changes, but also have several career changes. They need skills in resilience just to navigate those waters. Who we are should dare not be consumed and dictated by our work. There must be more to us than that. Then, our lives can have a harmony and a vibrancy that otherwise is impossible.

Take care of yourself. Who you are and who you're meant to be are so important. Be conscious of your selfhood; protect and nurture it. Don't let anyone or anything warp you. Overcome soul-sucking and soul-crushing forces. Nurture your integrity. Work is necessary and good, but work can also put you in the ground.

I've always taken pride in my work. Without having to claim that I was the best at anything, I have been able to claim that I did my best. A favorite way I put it is this: If I mow a yard or detail a car or sing a song, you can count on me doing my best. As a kid out of school in summer, I got to do my share of playing and some vacation time, but I worked a lot, too.

At my dad's store I learned quickly how to wait on customers and run the cash register (I remember the first $100 bill somebody handed me, which in 1971 went a *long* way), how to pump gas in all sorts of cars and trucks, how to sort returned glass Coke bottles, how to stock shelves, and more. It was a lively place, different every day, and I quickly took to it. Over time, I would take certain tasks upon myself, even without my dad asking me. It was because I took a sense of "ownership" in the place. For example, I dusted, organized, and restacked every item in the store. It was tedious work, often interrupted as I had to wait on customers, but the look of things pleased me. And, my dad liked it, too.

Beyond many hours of working as a "store boy," I did a lot of mowing and other work around our farm, plus mowing and bush-hogging jobs I picked up in the community surrounding our home and the store. I liked that, too. I've continued that commitment and ownership and pride and diligence in every job I've ever done. And, I've worked a lot of 14-hour days over the years. I've been happy and prideful in much of my work. I've also known what many others have known when the work wasn't only long and hard but also was wearyingly stressful due to difficult customers or management or economic difficulties. It's in these times that I've had to bring my best coping skills into their full array.

If you find yourself in these circumstances, that's what you have to do to not get taken down. It's important to stay ahead of difficult people and situations. And in maintaining integrity, it matters that you don't either "eat people alive" or steal and cheat or do embarrassing things to achieve success. On your way to the top, you first have to decide if you even need to go there and whether it's worth everything it takes to get there. Maybe you don't have to be all the way at the top. But, no matter how high you get, always pay up by "sending the elevator back down" for those at the bottom.

There's a lot to think about here. Again and again, when I've faced challenging times and difficult people , I've gained strength and perspective when I first made sure where I had my feet planted—that I was being fair, clear-minded, doing the right thing. Then, I had to take stock and remember who I am: I'm Jim, husband and father to three wonderful women, a friend of friends with character, church member/singer/deacon, civic contributor, and more. Then I could tip my hat and step back in and swing, look people in the eye, keep calm and centered, and go for what's true and best. The more I keep in touch with who I am and who I'm called to be, the more satisfying life gets.

Value your self-worth.

Most people interpret the meaning of self-worth in the traditional sense. But, if you're feeling beat up about your self-worth, you're probably looking for a lift, something to boost your feelings. Others will blow right by it because they already know they're the best thing since sliced bread, the bomb diggity, somebody everybody looks up to and wants to be like. Those with self-inflated or overinflated egos would do well to stop a minute and rethink. We'll do best if we learn to view our self-worth honestly and soberly. I promise this won't hurt a bit. Neither inflating nor deflating our self-worth serves us well.

I went through high school with a fellow who we all knew had the "big head." He was smart, athletic, tall, dark, and handsome. But oh, he knew it. I remember a bunch of us were waiting in line somewhere and, as usual, he was strutting his stuff right there in line. One of the fellows behind him in line got to having some fun mocking him. We were getting a kick out of it. He'd start to look our way, but we'd all act like nothing was going on. He'd turn back around, and the mimicking would resume. I'll never forget it. It also made an impression on me about not being too full of myself. I've seen the opposite, too.

I've known good, kind, hard-working people who didn't think enough of themselves. Many of us thought highly of them, but things they'd say and do revealed a low sense of self-worth. Me? I've had some moments where I needed a little humbling. And, I've had times when I didn't think enough of myself. I've been blessed by some really good people improving my perspective both ways.

Part of preserving our selfhood is realizing we're persons of worth. All of us have intrinsic value, apart from any accomplishments or social position or accumulated wealth. We all know people to whom we either look up or look down. The things people do that make them "bad" hopefully most of us don't want to do. As hard as it is to "be good" sometimes, over the long haul it proves easier, fulfilling, and happier for everybody.

As important as it is to do well, to do your best, to contribute and grow as a person, your self-worth doesn't come from fat bank accounts, marble entryways, diplomas on the wall, or athletic trophies. What you enter this world with and what you leave this world with are the same except for who you love, the memories you enjoy, the contributions you make, and the character you become. At some point, you have to learn to base your self-worth on these realities and on the things that really matter in life—wonderful things and wonderful people who help us when we encounter bad days and bad people.

I've been embarrassed at times at how I've allowed others to treat me—and when I started to believe them. I've dealt with some nasty, conniving people along the way. I never let them get me for too long, but I've had my days where they "got my goat." I wasn't cocky and arrogant but instead questioned myself at length as to whether they were right. Eventually, I confirmed for myself that these were indeed conniving people. But I also questioned if I could be at fault or undeserving or off-base or just plain wrong. I shook it out, did a lot of prayerful introspection, discussed it with wise friends, and came out on the other side wiser and tougher—and more sure of myself and my intrinsic self-worth.

There really are bullies in this world. Because of their warped understanding, stored-up anger, bitterness, and fear, they take things out on people. You can really get beat down by them. Many people suppress the bullying to some hidden inner storage unit; others try to eat or drink or shop it away.

These attempts at coping never work. Resist thoughtfully, shrewdly, coolly, and calmly, yet strongly! This is what I've done when I've been bullied, and it brought me out on the other side. There have been times when I awakened from the fog, realized what was happening, and even became ashamed that I'd believed the bullies and allowed them to put me down. I would ask myself: If the people I value most in life—my closest family and friends, and, yes, God—were hearing this stuff right now, were witnessing this abuse, would I be ashamed? So, why am I taking it now? This has encouraged me and put me in touch with my self-worth that I need to protect, and that strengthened my perspective in the moment.

Avoid self-centeredness.

We had a cat named Hope that lived 18 long years. If you'd asked her, she would have told you she was the center of the universe. You don't want to be like our cat. She thought everything was about her.

How about you? Are you self-centered and unaware? Let me urge some introspection and soul-searching.

As much as I love and enjoy people, in spite of many things I can point you to that I think are good, I also believe that we are the most self-centered society in the history of humankind. Don't let that reflect a sarcastic, fatalistic, pessimistic tone in me. But the evidence keeps mounting. Could you be part of the problem? It's easy to get sucked into thinking only about "me" and "mine" and "I want it now."

You see it in traffic: Let me through! I've got to go now! You see it in the throngs of people who have lots more than their folks had 40 years ago: They spend much of their waking hours feeding both the desire for more and the fear that somebody will take it away. You see it in various gatherings: The same people step forward to demand that things be done their way, at their time, and without consideration of what others may wish. It shows up in social struggles: The "haves" want what they have *and* what others have, yet fear that "others" will take something from them.

Self-centeredness shows up in myriad ways. Some of us will go to great lengths to cater to selfish people, no matter how miserable it makes us. I don't believe in catering to selfish friends or family members, much less in business or at community organizations or church or in politics! I know how to cater to customers, but there are things I'm willing to do and things I'm not. Call that a personal decision, and a business decision.

Now, I'll confess to dealing with some self-centeredness by playing what my daughters and I call "grocery store games" when we encounter an oblivious shopper. It's the man or woman who has the whole aisle blocked while searching for their item or having a long phone conversation. To break them out of their trance, I have a ploy: I know fully well that an item I want is on a shelf next to where the person is standing, but I look back at my daughters and ask loudly: "Is is this ketchup or that one there?" When that doesn't work, I'll just reach right over the shopper and take the item and then walk away—while he or she is still blissfully unaware that I've been there. (I'm glad for those people that I'm not a pickpocket or purse thief!) My daughters and I will walk away and have a good laugh—instead of becoming impatient and angry.

My point is that I've learned to not get angry, but instead to handle the self-centeredness of others with humor and wit—and sometimes mischief. The grocery store story is just one example of how selfish we can be. Other examples revolve around the things people insist they must have—and what they'll do to get them. When I hear people's list of "must-haves," I reflect on how inflated and embellished and exaggerated and unbelievable these things have become versus what people considered necessary, say, 40 years ago.

Let's become sensitive to our own symptoms of selfishness and self-centeredness. This alone would change the nature of many relationships. To borrow a phrase from my local church's covenant, learn "to live circumspectly." When my daughters and I walk away from another episode of our grocery store game, one of us inevitably mutters that we've just encountered another someone who hasn't learned "to live circumspectly." We need to develop "peripheral vision" so that we can be aware of others around us, and become selfless instead of selfish.

Are you doing okay in our current economy? Great. But realize that nobody is singly a "self-made" man or woman. If you've risen to the top, remember those at the bottom. Are you a successful owner or manager of your company? When you one day kick your feet up and relax and look back, will you be able to live with how you treated your people? Or, will you realize that you wrung more out of them than anyone should have to give?

In becoming selfless instead of selfish, we move from looking to give a handout (and maybe just making ourselves feel better) to becoming involved in structuring and remaking and advocating and even voting so that all boats truly rise with the waters. In becoming selfless instead of selfish, we move out of our comfort zone in our thinking and doing. We quit making excuses and explaining it all away so that we can help influence and cause lasting, good things to happen.

Seek to love and be loved.

Love is the best thing there is. Everybody deep down wants and needs love more than anything else. Love may get missed or pushed away or ignored, but when the wheels stop turning and the dust clears, it's love that we really need. As we look at taking care of our mind, spirit and emotions, love is an ingredient we dare not leave out.

Many people are "looking for love in all the wrong places." Others are running around with an axe, chopping down anything that sprouts up that might be love. Some have been hurt, embittered, or left behind, and cannot find or accept the love that may be offered to them. Still others are so caught up in striving for success and notoriety and sophistication that they have no time or interest in love. Do you have too much love in your life? We can have enough love, but we can never have too much. Love makes life worth living.

You may be too busy or important to know it, but you need to be loved and you need to give love. Love is the delight of a parent picking up a helpless baby out of its crib. Love is that baby smiling back. Love is making those first friends, and then more and more over a lifetime. Love is keeping many of those friends, and adding layers of moments and memories and blessings. Love is learning how to act in a friendship, in dating, in marriage, and as a family. Love is smiles and jokes and pats on the back as you come and go at work each day. Love is making sure you think about others and their needs beyond your own immediate understanding. Love is making decisions that are sometimes uncomfortable, that stretch you, that stretch your understanding, that stretch your heart, and that make you stretch out your arms and enlarge your circle.

Love is central to my understanding of faith as a Christian. It often makes me go against the grain, against the common Christian culture, and against many stereotypes in how all that plays out. According to the teachings of my faith, the most important thing of all is "to love God with all your heart, soul, mind and strength, and to love your neighbor as you love yourself." And all of this is in response to a God "who first loved us." Unfortunately, these must be the most overlooked and misunderstood yet wonderful concepts in the world.

One of my favorite stories is about the Grinch and how he has a big change of heart at the end of the story. In fact, his heart grows three sizes larger. Not only that, but the Grinch changes his behavior. He brings back all the toys he's stolen, and then gets invited to join in on the festivities. When he changes his thinking and feeling, his life changes radically. Love can do these things.

I have a dear friend who's half again as old as I. He has a tough, weathered exterior that has come with age and experience. Others near him, and I, joke about how he has to keep up his tough image—yet we know that he quietly does a lot of kind and benevolent things for a number of people around him.

I learned a lot about loving from even a young age, but 50 more years have taught me many more lessons. I believe they've made my heart grow, too. I can detail numerous things I see differently nowadays than I did in my youth, my 20s, 30s, even 40s. It seems I keep discovering new ways to stretch in love; new understandings about other people, about life, about the world, even about loving myself. These lessons in love continue to change me, not making me the greatest guy in the world, but certainly affecting me. You can't tell me you have too much love or that you love too much. See how many more sizes your heart can grow.

Seek help from within and without for depression and anxiety.

Failure to be loved by others or by oneself can result in depression and anxiety, which are evidenced in epidemic proportions in our society. If you are struggling with either or both, know you are not alone. There is help; there are ways out. While I feel that I've never been depressed, I've known numerous people who were. Some were diagnosed as depressed and some were not.

I have had my share of sad days, difficult times, times where I had to trudge through and persevere to happier times. I've also experienced my share of anxious times created by demanding, aggressive, confused, conniving, and just plain crazy people I've encountered in the work world. And, I might add, such encounters can lead many of us to have times of "trauma from drama" wherein we "overthink" and experience anxiety about what might happen next. I've thankfully learned some things from all these encounters that have helped me tremendously.

Depression and anxiety can compose a silent, invisible, heavy load—like a "dragging anchor." If you're carrying this load, you don't have to do it alone. Hold on to these suggestions for the turbulent times:

- Admit if you are down, worried, temporarily defeated.
- Don't compound the problem by reacting to others in ways you'll regret later.
- Attempt to deal with the actual causes of worry or anxiety or grief.
- Process the negativity in your life positively and healthfully, and head for higher ground.
- Make sure there is more to life than the obstacles you are facing.
- If you're facing a struggle at work, with health, or in relationships, don't leave room in your mind for the "cloud."
- Fill your life and your mind with fruitful engagements, relationships, thoughts, activities, and more that compose your life with good things.
- Leave the things and people that need to be "squeezed out."
- Muster the strength and resources to face certain people and situations head on: confront, resolve, then move on.

Apart from personal and physical tragedies that may not be overcome, there is hope, there is help, there are ways to happiness.

It's great to be strong: that's a good goal, physically and mentally. But in reality, there are times when we all need help. It's not a sign of weakness to get help with our troubles. By debriefing, ventilating, gaining perspective and enjoying support, we can be stronger than we would otherwise be. Our spouse may or may not be the person with whom to rehash each troubled day. The network may need to be expanded. There may be times we need the counsel of a professional. Also, we need to make sure that "rehashing" is never just griping and "reliving" what has bugged us. We need to make sure we're "going somewhere" as we discuss and sift through our troubles, so that we're working toward a new perspective and resolution.

Live with optimism and confidence.

In thinking about the downward, grinding forces in our lives, I think about the work of glaciers. Their size and movement and appearance fascinate us in photos, movies, and even up close and personal. Glaciers carve the places they move through on a slow but grand scale. They've become an even bigger deal in recent decades as climate change makes them melt and retreat faster than they should. When we joke about things moving at a glacial pace, that normally means really slow. Glaciers move downhill and then fall into a body of water. As they move, they grind and move surfaces with tremendous force.

My point is this: We can combat the downward, grinding forces we encounter in daily life so that we can be happier, freer, more at peace, stronger, and healthier. Here are some suggestions:

• Help yourself be strong. Get in touch with the fact that you were made to be strong in the face of life's challenges and challengers. While you won't succeed at everything and you won't win over everybody, you were meant for sunny days and health and happiness. That's what you can and should always gravitate toward. Tough times and difficult people don't last forever; you can get through them. Continually nurture your mental and spiritual and emotional strength, even as you simultaneously nurture your physical strength. The stronger your emotional intelligence, the better things will be. Learn from everything and everybody, and grow, grow, grow. Become "rock solid," so that the "glacial forces" of life cannot move you or grind you down.

• Be "light on your feet"—emotionally, mentally, and spiritually. Don't be weighed down by everything that can burden you. I once worked with individuals going through difficult times such as family breakups, deaths, and grief. I was grateful that I could be of help to them, but did not feel burdened by their problems. Someone who worked alongside me in these situations, however, was visibly wearied mentally and emotionally by taking on these people's burdens personally. In helping situations, for your own health and for your continued usefulness, you have to be alert to this. To avoid burnout and other difficulties, you can't feel every "bump in the road." Learn how to "float" over "irregularities" and changes and challenges. Develop "emotional suspension" to absorb the bumps in the road and not take everything so hard.

• Pay attention to what you're griping about on a regular basis, and learn to ask yourself if it's really a burden you need to take on. You don't have to fight every battle. I've heard it all my life: "let things roll off your back, like water off a duck." At times this ability can seem elusive, but we can and should learn to not stew on everything and relive the negativity; otherwise, things just seem worse. Don't collect burdens such as hurts and slights and insults and fears. Don't make a place in your mind to keep them and let them add up and fester. Free yourself of that stuff!

• Think about things, but don't overthink. I'm a thinker. Usually, that serves me well. I digest things, ponder them, savor good times and good things and good memories, analyze things and try to understand how they came about. I try to be thoughtful, considerate, and empathetic. I try to speak after thinking instead of speaking without thinking. In thinking, we can gain wisdom. But let's be careful about overthinking. When we overthink, we can come up with every internal scenario of "what could go wrong." To a point, that can serve us well by keeping us from being blindly optimistic. It can prepare us for what could happen, and those things that need some consideration. But overthinking becomes paralyzing when we become frozen in fear and inaction. Be considerate and take action that is smart, but realize you cannot control everything and that sometimes bad things will happen.

There can be times in life when we feel defeated, whipped, spent, trashed, demeaned, or not too happy with ourselves. If you haven't done any horrible things to others—murder, abuse, racism, or otherwise demeaning acts, for example—my first question to you would be, "Why are you so down on yourself?" That starting point helps to identify what needs to change.

As I said before, I've had my times in life where I had to trudge through, persevere, and struggle with real challenges, as well as some imaginary ones (overthinking!). I've met plenty of people who were downhearted and bleary-eyed. It takes more than a hearty hello and a word of cheer for deeply sad people. We have to identify reasons to hold our head high and see where the sun shines. No matter your circumstance, be aware that you are a person of worth and have something to offer to others and our world. Time is wasting. Every minute and every day ahead of you can be lived better than whatever you've faced before. Connect with the right people and resources and find the good in life and in your life. Live with optimism and confidence

We can be confident without being arrogant. Let's be kind enough to ourselves to step forward and say and do the good things that boost confidence as a byproduct. And, let us be sincere enough in introspection to avoid overconfidence, to avoid stubbornness, to avoid arrogance, to steer clear of being a big-headed fool. Having the clarity to keep our balance is one of the best things we could hope to achieve in life. Make the effort!

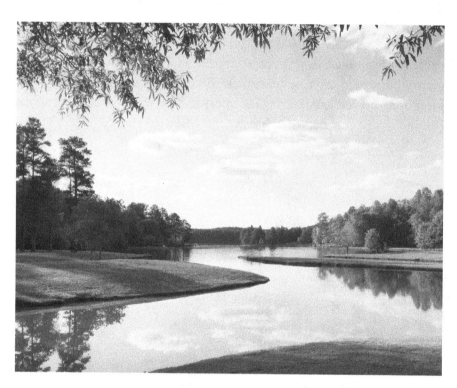

Starting from a mindset of love (or not) affects all relationships.

Chapter 3

Take Care of Your Relationships

Who you are is what you bring to the table. I remember my first friends in school. I got to skip kindergarten and went right to first grade, and there they were. There were a few characters I remember to this day.

I remember the first crush I had. I went all the way through school in my hometown with her. Another first friend passed away years ago. Another friend I remember from those first days in school and have always held in high regard still lives in my hometown and is now my mother's general practitioner. I remember being glad to see everybody at school every day, unless they proved otherwise. But I don't remember much of that. I did know that nobody had anything to fear from me. It's always been that way.

I've awakened each day prepared to be a friend, if that was acceptable. At times I've grieved when it wasn't. Eventually, I learned that not everybody shared my agenda. But I've had and still have many wonderful friends. And, I keep on making them. My understanding of who I am has not substantially changed over time. I've often said that I get up every day to love people, have adventures, do the best I can to help my world, and make a living.

What do you bring to the world every day? What would people honestly say about you?

Acknowledge your family of origin.

As a boy, I sometimes wondered how I was born to the parents I had. It wasn't that I had any gripes about it, just how I ended up with them instead of somebody else. What if I'd been born a black girl in Mississippi or Nigeria? Why wasn't I born Robin Roberts, the *Good Morning America* anchor of similar age?

Who is in your family and what those people are like and how they treat each other affect many things. Realizing you could have been born somebody else in a different place ought to make you have compassion for people from different places. As a parent, and now as a grandparent, I've been cognizant that I've not only wanted to love my children very much, but I've also wanted to help them discover much about living and relationships. I've also wanted to do my darnedest to make sure they didn't have to overcome any dynamics from me.

Many people I've met have damage, hurts, baggage, and more from their family of origin. If these are not factors you've had to overcome, then be grateful. But many people have things to work around, grapple with from their family. Many aren't aware of how all this affects their personality, how they behave, and how they approach life. Becoming aware—whether good, bad, or neither—helps to increase our ability to be objective, to understand how we see things and hopefully to improve how we respond to them. It can be enlightening!

Start with a mindset of love.

Love or lack of it affects all relationships. Let's learn to love our families of origin, as they are. For some people, that may take some processing, but it can be done. The families we create, let's love them; otherwise, why should we have them? Before that, in our friendships and dating relationships, let's apply love and see how much better those relationships go.

Love (instead of something lesser, such as infatuation, lust, convenience, and prestige that bring people together) proves itself in genuine affection and care. Love needs to happen at work, by loving and respecting ourselves as we walk in every morning, by working hard to offer our highest quality each day, by loving the people we work with—no matter how easy or difficult that is. Love should determine how we respond to the people who wait on us in restaurants, who change the linens at the hotel where we stay, and a host of other moments. In the board room, in the office, with our students, with our clients, whoever we work with, even as we conduct business, how we go about it should be determined by love.

If love is much more than just fluff and trite sayings, the nature of our relationships will have a different, better, higher quality. We should try for this more and more. Love will change how we see the world each day.

Accept family dynamics.

A family we love and that loves us is a tremendous gift. But not everyone has that, so "family" gets found in different and creative ways sometimes. A loving family is built one day at a time, one exchange at a time, one challenge at a time, one good experience at a time. We've got to want such a bond, and nurture it all the time. The more we put in, the more we get. Of course, there are things beyond our control.

We cannot determine the behavior of others in the mix; we can only respond to their behavior. It requires regular input and sometimes tactical discussions to establish healthy structures and ways of relating. But it's worth the effort. Like flowers in a garden, we have to tend and nurture relationships often. Then, they'll bloom in ways that make us proud. This doesn't happen overnight, but unfolds one moment into one day into years of time.

Whatever yours is like, respond well to your family. If your family of origin was fun and loving, give thanks! You have been given something that is more the exception than the norm. If your family was fun and loving, then learn how to keep it going. Keep the tradition. Enjoy and relish the moments with that good, loving family. Welcome newcomers into that family, and make them keep the code! If you don't have a fun and loving family of origin, work to overcome the negative stuff.

Instead of being victimized, wounded, and bitter because of tough family dynamics, try to understand and identify what wasn't workable or desirable. Then, respond well to negative dynamics and difficult people in your family. Seek to have a loving relationship with those persons. Learn and practice forgiveness, if nothing else, to free yourself from the bad things that have happened. Sometimes you may have to articulate and set limits within those family dynamics. You may find moments when you have to assert yourself and make clear where you stand on an issue.

I've long said that I don't care to cater to difficult people and drama people. As cooperative as I can be, I don't like to "plow around" such people. Rightly or not, I've been told repeatedly that I have "the patience of Job." I'll take that endorsement! But I've found that in my best moments I also have become assertive at the right time and said what needed to be said. This is a healthier alternative to letting things fester, to letting everybody be miserable around each other for years, to becoming passive-aggressive and hinting around about things that are irritating.

Strive for the best for you and your family, the one you have and the one you want.

Nurture the best possible relationships with family members.

Nurture your relationships with your parents as best you can. If relationships with them are comfortable and free-flowing, then share life's daily experiences with them. If not, share what you can and connect where you can. Spend time with your parents when possible. Call them. Take some extra effort to stay connected. Time passes and life gets away from you, so putting it off usually is a mistake. If things are difficult, then work to gain an understanding of what's difficult, and respond to it as positively and constructively as possible. Work to accumulate good memories together and see how these can transform relationships. Allow yourself to forgive, to be free, and to heal. Be better to your parents than they were to you. You're responsible for what you do, not what they do. Gain satisfaction in that.

I'm glad my daughters are close. My wife and I have threatened them with what we'd do if they weren't! When siblings enjoy each other throughout life, it's a blessing to both them and their parents. I love to see siblings who are close in adulthood, who keep in touch, who laugh comfortably together, who do things together when they can. Invest in that. For those who aren't close or even estranged, seek to forgive, to reconcile, to rebuild the relationship, to have good experiences together. If circumstances prevent that, just do the best you can—that's what you're responsible for.

I've been to many happy weddings. Unfortunately, too many of those didn't last. I'm beyond happy to say that my wife and I have more than 35 happy years of marriage to celebrate. Everybody who knows us knows we're close. We were quickly engaged after meeting at age 19, but waited till we were 21 and a week out of college to get married. The rest is history. Gray hair is the only thing that has changed about her, and she's still fascinating to me. I'd say we still have that dating attitude about us, but better than that with time and experience and years of bonding. Even during the years we were raising our children, we made time for each other. Our children saw us laughing and talking together about everything, serious and not so serious. Here are some suggestions I have for nurturing relationships with our spouses:

- Never stop finding delight in the person you love the most.
- Nurture what delighted you initially to bloom and grow.
- Stack up more good moments than bad.
- Watch it when you're tired and weary.
- Don't let your mood determine the quality of your relationship.
- Don't let whatever bugs you, angers you, or needs forgiving stack up and fester.
- Watch what you're sarcastic about; sarcasm often reveals underlying anger.
- Be true to your vows, especially that part about "to love and to cherish."
- Be true to each other.
- Don't cheat; don't even develop a wandering eye.

(Wandering eyes should set off a warning that something needs to be dealt with—quickly and seriously. Before you head toward that phrase "something about him/her has changed," take steps to deal constructively with issues and to build intimacy and delight with each other. Many of the answers to the troubles that couples have are rooted in failing to take care of themselves. For example, many couples get tired personally and tired of each other. They need rest and restoration, and the sooner the better.)

Before my wife and I had children, a sizable number of youngish parents told us in various ways things that made us wonder why they had children at all. We kept hearing about how life would change, about all the things we wouldn't be able to do or to afford, and basically how inconvenient children would be. Now, I think most of these people loved their children; they were just not having as much fun as they could. Here are some suggestions I have regarding parenting:

- Be realistic before having children. They aren't like adopting puppies (or maybe they are). They're expensive. They require lots of attention. Prepare for them.
- Enjoy your children. Don't turn them into overachievers. Enjoy the little things and the simple moments, especially in nature.
- Spend a lifetime sharing life with your children, regardless of their age. There's much to discover together.

Every now and then, something we see triggers the conversation, and my wife and I will start laughing and agree that we'd hate to be out in the dating world now. Thankfully, we'd want to meet each other again. But frankly, most of what I see out there doesn't appeal. (They might say the same for me!) If I had it to do all over again, I don't know that I would approach dating differently. I'd look for someone attractive, good, kind, smart, thoughtful, thinking, and unselfish. I would invest time in building and nurturing the relationship. In regards to this principle, I would suggest to couples:

• Spend lots of time talking about and exploring what matters to both of you.
• Major on more substantive things than how you spend money on each other.
• Notice what makes you uncomfortable and causes conflict, and work at resolving those issues satisfactorily and constructively.

I don't think I have much non-traditional family, but I have many friends who are in non-traditional families. I'm way past thinking these are strange or different. I think they're wonderful. Not everyone grew up living like Ozzie and Harriet. Love and circumstances pull people together in all sorts of family arrangements that are family for them. Non-traditional families share a big need in common with traditional families: lots of love within the family, and lots of love from without. That love will always need nurturing and feeding. Our support networks need set no limits. Let's get longer arms to reach out further around us in love.

Nurture relationships with friends.

I've never had and can't have too many friends! I'll always keep making friends. Several years ago, I met a couple who would become wonderful friends. On a follow-up call to the man, I didn't hesitate. I went right for "the close." I pointed out several things I noted that we had in common. And I said that I hoped we could "continue the conversation." Thankfully, he said, "Well, you just consider yourself my buddy." It all started there, and several years of good experiences and hours of conversations have ensued. I treasure the friendship of this couple. It matters to me.

Again, I don't need to keep stats on how many friends I have or how many I have versus other people. Being popular can be very different from having good friends. A few good friends are always more valuable than just knowing a bunch of people.

I've achieved "friends with character." I'd thought about this idea, but last year my son-in-law articulated it after having met yet another of my cherished friends. Among my friends in whom I most delight, I do have quite a lineup of "friends with character." They have proven to be great friends who care sincerely, with whom I've shared life's events, and whom I appreciate for their own general character. But also, these friends are truly "characters" themselves, often funny, yes, but also friends who make quite a contribution wherever they are. These friends with character aren't boring; they're interesting people with something going on in their lives and in their minds. I'm glad I know them.

Friends should never drain you. Friends give; they never take away. I've had friends who were a drain, and I've certainly observed "friends" who were a drain. They were parasitic, there for their own needs instead of seeking a "symbiotic," mutual, reciprocal relationship. Being around people like these is tiring. Give and take: that's what friends are for. Just the joy of being together, sharing experiences, laughing together, helping each other, being there in the moments of life: that's what friends are for. Being pulled into drama, catering to silly or emotional spider webs, keeping up with the Joneses: that's not what friends are for.

You do find out who your friends are. If you live long enough, you'll go through times when your real friends prove themselves. Hopefully we can prove to others that we're that kind of friend, too. It's great to develop dear friends in life who you delight in hearing from, with whom you laugh for hours, and who are there when there's sadness. Cherish those friendships. And, go surprise someone soon and be a friend they didn't even realize they had.

What's great is to have friends you just enjoy for years and have in case you need them—and end up never needing them. If you can go through life and just be great friends and have good times, that's fantastic. But most of us experience at least once in our lifetime when we need our friends. Then, it's a treasure to find out who they are. Cherish their support. Those who prove to not be friends, who are not caring and supportive, just let them go. Pay attention to those who turn out to be true friends.

Nurture relationships in the workplace.

If you're an employer, there are times when it's really good to be the boss—and there are times when it's really bad. One day behind the counter at my dad's store, when I was maybe no more than 11 years old, I remember pondering how that business was our place and yet every day we let all these people come in. I quickly learned to say to every customer I waited on: "Thank you" and "Come back."

If you own a business, you want people coming in, spending money, and coming back. As long as they do, that's good. You also want workers who make them want to come back, workers who you have trained in how you want things done (or maybe discovered that they do even better than you'd imagined) and who make your life better. Ask yourself:

• Do I make the lives of my employees better?
• Do I foster respect from my employees and in return get "natural respect"?
• Do I make it possible for them to take ownership in the company and pride in their work?
• Could I discover some secrets from satisfied workers and customers?

If you're a leader of any type of organization, you shoulder the challenges and opportunities of leading those with whom you work. The long-term success of doing business stems from how you manage and work with people. I enjoy many good exchanges at businesses I patronize. I am very loyal at these where I get sincere, competent, welcoming service. But I've exited businesses where I've had subpar experiences, all of which I attribute to poor management.

It's evident these days that many employees receive little or no training and supervision in the basics of their job and whatever customer service they provide. The only thing many employees know is when they start work and when they get off work. Many managers and owners would say this is because it's hard to get good help. But much of the problem stems from managerial failure to build a culture that requires excellence.

When I can walk into our local grocery stores and know better where things are than the employees I've been seeing there for a while, someone needs training. When I've dealt with real estate transactions handling clients' most precious and expensive possessions, it becomes evident that much of the industry needs training in ethics, professionalism, how to communicate in something more than just texts, location and its big-picture and little-picture implications, and a host of other subjects.

Whether it's in college business classes or in continuing ed classes or in Chamber of Commerce seminars or in training opportunities, the instruction should be about developing a corporate culture fitting to the company or organization. Otherwise, folks just work the register and mutter to each other, "What time do you go on break?" And too many of them just give their time, then go home to drink it off and try and cope with their bosses, coworkers, and "the public." I'm always delighted by companies and organizations that decide there's a better way.

When it comes to employees, everywhere I've worked I could name for you good coworkers. Some of them I still keep up with across the years and miles. It's good to "have each other's back," to build bonds of friendship and comradeship, to become a "well-oiled machine," and more. Sometimes I walk into an office or business and see the evidence of this. On the other hand, there are other offices and stores where dread and apathy fill each Monday, where conflict and fear and anger prevail, where people grind it out year after year and drug it off each weekend, and where strategizing about retirement is about "whether I can stand it that long." That's no way to live. So, as an employee:

- Learn to live with your fellow employees and the bosses.
- If you land in a wonderful situation, count yourself fortunate.
- Learn how to work with the myriad personalities within your company and with your customers.
- Make your own mark, your own way in the company.
- Take ownership in your company.

Maybe it was because I grew up in a family-owned business, maybe it was just how I came to see things, but one thing that has helped me through the years is a sense of ownership. Wherever I've worked over the years, I've bought in and made it my own. I'm not saying I was the best, but I could say I always gave it my best. Even though I didn't own the place, I owned the place! Not that I was asserting to be top dog, but I devoted myself to doing my job the best I knew how and to be aware beyond my "area."

Having a sense of ownership doesn't mean you start poking your nose into how everybody does their job or that you watch the clock to see if they're earning their keep or just there taking up space. It means you mentally own the place, maybe with the benefit of not having to worry about "overhead." It means you want things to run their best, look their best, go their best. It means you work hard. And, it means you can look back with satisfaction at a job well done. You're taking care of yourself when you take care of where you work.

My attitude about ownership goes back to my formative experiences. I've mowed yards and pastures since I was 10 years old. I've never finished mowing that I didn't stop at least once to look back over a field or lawn to see if I missed a spot or just to take satisfaction in how it looked. Over the years I've enjoyed waxing our cars, my bikes, and other vehicles frequently. I like the results. And every time when I'm done, I'll stop and look to see if I missed a spot, and just enjoy the satisfaction of it all—maybe eight times! That's ownership. Go to work that way and come home happier.

Learn to work with all types of people.

In our work we may have to deal with tough customers, tough bosses, and tough coworkers. One of the first things you need to learn about the workplace, like most everywhere else: There's almost always at least one bad apple in the bunch. Not everybody will be glad to see you on your first day of work: let's hope the boss isn't one of those. There's the initial fitting in that you have to do, and then it all evolves from there. Hopefully, you get a good welcome and get shown "your place" and you get started. Let's hope things go well and you're off to a good start. As time passes, you can begin to fit in and even begin to prove yourself. But remember:

- Don't strut around like a know-it-all, but instead, lean toward acting like you don't know as much as you do.
- Work hard at learning everything you can, especially at first. You have to "master the craft" before you can be a master at the craft.
- Strive to become an "essential employee," one the company cannot do without and who gains long-term respect and appreciation.

What do people gather from you every day at work? It's always been my practice and habit to walk in and greet anybody I see with a sincere smile. That's usually what I'm feeling inside. I have total disregard for whether you're a morning person or not or in a good mood or not. That doesn't mean I bounce all over everybody like Tigger or force some kind of fake enthusiasm, but I do walk in glad to see folks before taking care of business. It's kind of like the "rally" a pack of wolves have before trotting off to hunt.

When I've been a manager, I've counseled employees that I didn't ever want to see them walking in with "a knot in their gut" over anything or anybody they were dealing with. And, if so, they needed to get with me right away and talk about it and see what we could do. If more managers/bosses did that, companies and organizations would be much healthier and more productive, stress and health problems would be lessened, and we'd have a happier world.

Once we get in our "office," it's important to get to the tasks of the day, doing what we do to our very best, while still creating a mutually motivating environment. Whether we are the boss or not, what we say and do and how we go about it should motivate instead of demotivate, encourage instead of discourage, and cooperate instead of compete. We need to ask ourselves:

- Could I be the problem?
- Am I lazy and unmotivated and just watching the clock?
- Am I using my computer for things unrelated to my job?
- Can others depend on me?
- Am I just in the way?
- Am I a grumpy person?
- Is everybody having to work around me?
- Am I always the one in a bad mood?
- Am I a drama queen or drama king?

These are questions that many fellow workers would like for their bosses and coworkers to grapple with. Maybe it's time for you to do that. Transform how you fit in and contribute at work by answering these questions honestly and seriously. Let's start working better.

Identify your organizational role.

Some of us have our "appointed duty" in life. You may know what yours is. I've been told repeatedly that my duty has been to "steady the boat." It's not a job I signed up for, but yes, that has seemed to be my thing. At work, in organizations, and in other circles, I've had to step up and be the voice of reason—the one who kept his cool, the one who negotiated to a workable end, the one who helped fix the wounded. Sometimes it's messy, sometimes it's scary, sometimes it's bumfuzzling at what people can do to each other. Sometimes I've had to be the mediator between the hothead and everybody else. Let's just say a series of life's events over the years led me to this role—again, without my volunteering.

Remember, I wanted to be a wolf biologist—you know, hidden out behind a rock somewhere in the great Northwest without another soul around, trying to be quiet and observe an elusive, cunning, alert, wildest of wild creatures. Instead, I ended up juggling people. But I've found again and again that somebody's got to do it, and repeatedly it's fallen to me.

I've never liked to see conflict take its course without efforts at reconciling, stabilizing, healing, correcting the situation if possible. I've been most satisfied in those moments when I've been willing to "kick the can" in another direction when most everybody wanted to appease or cater to the bully. It's not what I get up to do any morning, but when necessary, yeah, let's go. In addition to my role of steadying the boat, I'm also good at steering from the back of the boat.

Several years ago, a civic club I was in got involved in our local dragon boat races. My wife and I had fun getting in on that, both the group practices and the actual competition. There were a couple of hairy, funny moments when some big fellows decided to swap sides of the boat in the middle of the lake. I ended up being the steerer for our boat—from the back—and I enjoyed it.

I've thought back on that fun experience numerous times as I've been in meetings and negotiations and even when helping clients, and found myself steering from the back. It can be done, and sometimes that's the most effective place from which to steer. One of the good things about steering from the back is that people may forget you're back there, thinking they're doing all the deciding and the steering when actually you are—or, you're at least keeping things on course. More seriously, I've found that if people can shake out what they're considering up front, I can follow behind and help steer things better while allowing them to retain a sense of ownership in what we're doing. People rarely take to being led where they don't want to go. There's an art to steering from the back—and a whole different thing than being a backseat driver!

Learn to get along with the boss.

It's been said that everyone has a boss, especially unless you own the company or are mega wealthy. I've never been one to fear bosses, but I have had to deal with them. Most of my bosses have been at least pretty good, but some have been terrible: They kept everybody upset and caused themselves problems due to the repercussions of their own behavior.

What have your experiences been like with your bosses? Bosses, how are you doing? It matters. Many bosses make things much harder than they have to be.

Good or bad, you relate to the boss. You deal with the boss either well or poorly, or you look in the mirror at the boss. I've never been one to "kiss up" to the boss nor fear the boss. Instead, I've sought every day to be an asset to the boss, with the goal of proving to be an essential employee the boss just had to have. I've tried to continually learn as much as possible at my job, seeking to improve on what I've done. After that, I want to be as friendly as is doable with the boss, which of course depends on the personalities involved.

Good bosses enable employees to do their very best by creating a climate that makes that possible. They set high expectations and standards, live up to those standards themselves, and celebrate the achievements. Bosses should be enablers, not disabling critics. They should not be in the way, but should show the way. Unfortunately, bosses too often are the problems instead of the enablers.

Perhaps my worst boss ever was just a real tyrant. I'd been working at my job a while and had generally proven myself to him and didn't usually get that much trouble. But day after day, "reports" would start floating up to me, warning me to watch out because he was in a bad mood. My reply would be, "And . . .?" That was my way of making clear that moods were not a factor to me. I was about the work and the way we did it.

I don't like dealing with moods. I'm fine with working through the rough issues, as long as we deal with them productively and constructively. I'm not into chewing up people just because I can't cope or can't figure out anything else better. I've never been into "kicking the dog."

One time, another department head came to me demanding to ram something through that just wasn't workable. When I resisted him, he said, "Well you know, s___ runs downhill." Unflinching, I said, "And it stops right here with me." I negotiated with him about what we could do without ruining everything else we already had going. It was, I admit, a difficult workplace culture to endure.

Sometimes you have to decide how much you can endure in the workplace. Good bosses work hard to make sure it's a positive environment.

Strive to be an indispensable employee.

Thinking back to everywhere I've worked, even now I can remember who was indispensable. Management may or may not have agreed with my picks, but I'm pretty sure of them. The "essential employees" were people we needed every day. We could count on them; they got things done. Under the best circumstances, these were people of tenure who didn't come and go. Smart management would make sure they stayed. They were competent, hard-working, time-proven people. So, how can you be an indispensable, essential employee?

- Show up every day, on time and then some.
- Find joy and satisfaction and pride in your work.
- Be curious enough to learn new things.
- Don't grumble without some intent and direction.
- Work constructively, whether things are going well or not.
- Don't become hampered or dysfunctional just because things around you are going crazy.
- Work for and be responsible for yourself: make a statement about who you are by doing your best.
- Don't compound an excruciating time by adding to the problems.
- Be smart: avoid the gossip and griping that go on when things or individuals get out of hand.
- If you must discuss something, do it carefully and quietly; focus on the issues.
- Avoid power plays, but know when to confront or to leave.

Power plays rarely work. People in distress at work often dream of planning a coup, taking over, making needed change, ousting a leader. People in power at work sometimes devise power plays to put people in their place, to make a big sweeping change, or to surge ahead of the competition. Usually, the only people who get moved by power plays are the employees; for employers, the mission of the company isn't the motivator, but power is. Either way, there's almost always a high employee price that gets paid, and usually nobody involved likes that in the end.

When dealing with power plays, employees must look for ways to deal productively and constructively with issues, or else make a bold move such as confronting or leaving.

To confront problem people above you or below you at work, build as much stock as possible by first working hard, investing work and interest in the company, and by proving typically unflappable and peaceful. Being a drama queen or king doesn't set you up to be able to speak to issues when they arise. Prove your mettle, and save up influence for a rainy day—and hope it never comes. If it does come, don't confront when you're hotheaded. Sloppy, out-of-control showdowns usually turn into train wrecks. My most successful confrontations came after I let some dust settle, gathered my talking points, closed a door, didn't sit down, laid the cards on the table, and made clear my position and intention—and my wish to continue to be essential.

Sometimes confrontation doesn't work out. You need to think ahead what you might do. How do you decide when you need to take care of yourself and make a change? How do you decide when to go?

There is no exact formula for deciding when to make a necessary move and leave a job that is unworkable. Factors such as financial obligations, the current economic state, and more should be considered. In deciding to move on, it is advisable to have a next job to go to! But there are those of us who have "reinvented ourselves" more than once. It requires a lot of forethought and boldness and hard work, but sometimes the cost of staying in an unhealthy situation truly outweighs the risk of moving on. There can be life beyond the life you know now that is stuck between a rock and a hard place. You have to decide whether to stay or to go. Whichever you do, do it well.

Learn how to deal with customers.

Growing up in a store, as I did, teaches you to know your customers. Everybody can understand about having customers in a country store/convenience store. But honestly, no matter your line of work, you either have customers or you're out of business. Doctors need patients, attorneys need clients, schools need supportive parents, writers need readers, singers need concert-goers— you get the idea. Know who are your customers.

Realize what you have to offer your customers. Whatever your line of business, it has to match up with the customers you are serving. Over the years, if you watch, you'll notice businesses come and go. Banks run into this all the time. Would-be business owners approach a bank, asking for a business loan. When the bank asks for their business plan, they don't have one. So, the bank turns them down—or, they should. Sometimes they get the loan, and all too soon the business fails. If the business doesn't line up with the customers' wishes, there's no line of customers.

We usually want more customers, but sometimes a business has to decide its limitations—how many customers it can serve, maybe what is its niche— so that it can focus and be most effective. Still, the desired outcome is more output versus input, profit over cost. You have to realize what you cannot do for your customers without fighting them about it. Admit there's some things you're not good at and then focus on what you do best.

Sometimes you have to lose/fire customers. This perhaps has been one of the hardest lessons for me in business. I would blame myself, even though I'd been supremely patient and had bent over backwards. I believed what the customers said about me, even if it wasn't so. I worried and grappled about what I should do better and how I would learn to do so. Then, reality set in.

I was making myself sick trying to satisfy the unsatisfiable. I realized: these people weren't happy before we started, they're not happy now, and they probably won't be happy at the next place they stop. I finally learned to make a business decision and fire some customers. I've realized that I can take care of all the great customers and even the average ones 10 at a time instead of trying to make one dysfunctional customer happy—which is impossible. I've learned to identify those types early on and pass on their business. It's a decision that's paid off every time I've made it!

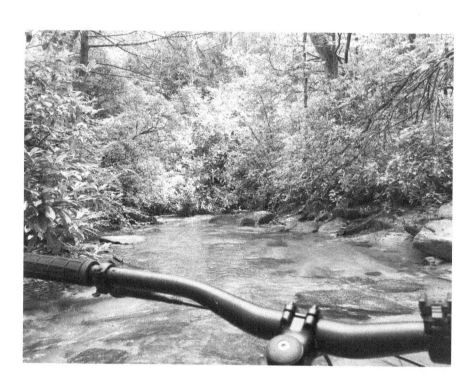

Sometimes we have to make decisions and take action.

Chapter 4

Take Care of Your Community

I love the opening scene in John Wayne's classic western, *Big Jake*, where he's watching a scene down below that he's tempted to get involved in. He pulls back from his rifle sight and says, no, I'm not gonna do it. He talks to himself about not getting in somebody else's business, even if it involves preventing a hanging. But then they shove the little boy down whose Dad is apparently about to be hanged. "Oh, why'd they have to go and do that?" John Wayne rides down and sticks his nose "in somebody else's business."

We're all taught from an early age to mind our own business. Much of the time, that is good instruction. We should live in peace with our neighbors, and that often means minding our own business. We don't usually stroll over and tell our neighbors how to cut their grass. But sometimes we may have to offer to help! And there are times when we can no longer be silent. There are times when we need to speak up, even if we are in the minority opinion.

A state of peace and quiet is precious. We all talk about wanting it. There's even a real estate concept and law centered around peace and quiet. We want to be left alone. We often say we want a vacation for some peace and quiet away from the rush and stress and demands of our jobs. So, we pay big money, load up the car, and drive long distances to the resort where everybody else is going and where there's all sorts of entertainment and noise so that we can have some peace and quiet. Then we cram everything and us back in the car and drive back in all that crazy traffic, and still long for peace and quiet. Are we missing something here?

Back home, we treasure peace and quiet. But we're gone somewhere all the time, and our neighbors' dog barks 24/7, and we watch real action on TV or videos. Peace and quiet! Yeah, we want that. Well, for my favorite version of peace and quiet, you'll find me on a big rock in the middle of a mountain stream in my favorite corner of the world—that is, if I can get across Atlanta.

Know when to involve yourself.

It seems every neighborhood has a busybody, a nosy neighbor, somebody who's minding everybody else's business. We once bought a home that had previously been owned by a nosy neighbor. How did we know that? The neighbors told us! I tried to assure them right away that things would be different with us.

Have you ever encountered a busybody? Ever had somebody nosing into your business? My wife's folks used to have a nosy neighbor. Every new thing that they ever acquired, the nosy neighbor would come over and inquire, even asking how much they paid. Some things are not our business, but some things we cannot afford to leave alone.

When the neighbors down the street let their grass grow a foot tall month after month (and it's not farm country), at some point it becomes a matter for you. It affects your home's value. We used to live on a cul-de-sac with some of the nicest neighbors you could imagine. But a couple of those neighbors were slack about mowing their yards. When they would go on vacation, while I was mowing our yard, I'd just ease over and mow their yard, too. They'd come home and see it mowed, find out I did it, and thank me profusely! I was glad they liked it, but they didn't know I was doing it for me.

Over the years in real estate, especially back during the Great Recession, I counseled people again and again to mow the yard of that foreclosure next door to protect their own investment. There are other issues that come up among neighbors. If your neighbor is making meth, it's an issue for you. If the dog next door jumps the fence and threatens visitors to your home, it's an issue for you. If the neighbors are fighting, it can be an issue for you.

Some years ago, my wife and I helped an abused woman and her children move to a shelter in the middle of the night. It had become our business. We couldn't ignore her problem. Adulthood means that sometimes we have to take action even when part of us wants to ignore and run away from the issue.

Pay attention to location.

Years of experience in real estate have proved to me how true is the adage "location, location, location." It's the most important factor in real estate, but also one of the most overlooked. People know it, yet they forget it. They get caught up in other factors (new construction, new appliances, three-car garage). I counseled all my clients, buyers and sellers alike, to never overlook location.

There's "macro location," such as the country club or amenities versus the highway. And, there's "micro location," such as the low side of the street versus the high side or a flat lot versus an overly steep lot. Where home is for you is more than "garage door up, garage door down." The "what" and "who" around your home are important. And as much as ever before, we need to get to know our neighbors.

Recently one of my neighbors came over and sat in the chair beside me on my porch while I was talking on the phone. I motioned him on in and wrapped up my call as quickly as possible, then we had a nice chat. I enjoy speaking to several of my neighbors regularly and warmly. But even after 15 years in our home, I've got neighbors as close as three houses away whom I've never met, who hardly ever come out of their home.

Grow roots where you live.

How long have you lived in your current home? Has it been more than a few weeks? Planning to stay for some time? If you haven't already, you need to grow roots in your community. And you might as well have fun while doing that. I have for years.

Get to know people. Get out. Get around. Hang back and observe and listen. Listen to who says what. Listen to how they say it. Read the local newspapers, and read between the lines. Don't believe everything you read and hear. Discern. Start to figure out where you want to fit in. As much as you want, find an organization or two or three with which to be involved. Give time to something that actually matters and that truly betters our world. I've done that for half my life now, and it's helped me so much.

There's a well-known episode of the *Andy Griffith Show* where a stranger moves to town. The term stranger was appropriate for this fellow, because he quickly made folks uncomfortable. As he mixed and mingled, it became evident that this newcomer knew all sorts of intimate details about everybody. They got scared. In the end, it all finally made sense, and people were relieved: The newcomer had been subscribing to and reading the local newspaper for some time prior to moving to town. He'd done his homework!

Look for opportunities that fit you.

After moving into a community, as soon as possible, find a place that fits you to express your religious commitments. "Missional involvement" should offer you somewhere to meet a genuine need or two in your area. Akin to that, there should be at least one cause you might be involved in. As much as my dad has always been appreciated back in my hometown, he never was a community-oriented man. He had his place, but it all revolved around his business. Frankly, he worked such long hours, there was no time for anything else. He missed out on the fun and fulfillment I've enjoyed in community involvements. But, then, back at Greenway Grocery, he was at the center of that community.

Several years ago I mused with my dad that, if an unknown uncle bequeathed me millions of dollars and I no longer had to work, or if I could retire tomorrow, I would—and I listed for him a litany of things I'd do. He looked at me like I was smoking crack. He just couldn't fathom what I'd described. Like I tell folks often, when I retire I won't sit and watch reruns of *The Price Is Right*. Honestly, between everything there is to be interested in, with more books to read than there is time, with bikes to ride, hikes to take, songs to sing, places to go, people to know and laugh with and worship with and be involved with, and needs to be met, I'm quite sure I'll never be bored. God, help that be so.

Make connections with the place and people.

I love maps. I've got maps tacked up in my garage, I've got maps stuck away in the door pocket of my car, and yes, I'm often studying Google maps. I like to see where everything is in relation to everything else. I tell everybody that one of the benefits of riding bicycles is that you get a more intimate knowledge of places. You slow down and see things you wouldn't see in a car. So, you, too, over time, learn what is where in communities and then learn why it's there and how that affects the people around it. Walk the streets at different times, especially on a quiet Sunday afternoon, and learn every dog and bush and fire hydrant. It'll change your view.

Most of us live busy lives. We may or may not be accomplishing much in those busy lives, but we're busy. Maybe it's time we mixed it up a little more. We get into a routine. That routine often involves "cocoons" and "silos."

I don't mean folks who are helping butterflies spread and who work on dairy farms. I'm referring to how we get in our cars (cocoons) and just live our 9-5 lives with people who look like us and dress like us (silos). This possible overstatement doesn't get as much good done as we actually wish. In a time when we have more ways to communicate quickly than ever (phone, text, social media, etc.), we're more disconnected than ever.

People are distrustful of each other. People are angry about everything under the sun. People are conflicting over everything imaginable. Some of our cocooning and siloing causes this. I get it. The answer is in connecting and mixing it up, and maybe we need you in the mix. Smile, wave, and have conversations. Get to know the folks in your town, or at least in your part of town. Get involved in the life of your town and help in some way. Connect and reconnect. Many people are longing for some of that small-town atmosphere and what made it that way.

So, you're 28, just a few years out of school, in debt, starting a career and I'm telling you to be a solid citizen. Or, you're 43, commuting every day, long hours, and here I go telling you to be "Citizen of the Year." We all have our limitations. But decide how you want to live and what you want out of your town. Don't just give up. Don't become cynical and sarcastic. Don't become Archie Bunker. Find ways to connect. Maybe reorganize your life a little, to make possible the things you want deep down inside.

Recently I called a friend who lives three hours away and told him I would be in his area in a couple weeks. I could have just left him alone, imagined he was too busy, but I called. We made plans to get together. Back home, some would say I've been too involved, considering my work schedules all these years. Maybe at times, that's been true. But I plan to continue as much involvement as I should, because I want to be a giver, not just a taker. So, that involves connecting, deciding, caring, getting involved, whatever it takes. Things could look better if we'd all lend a hand.

Identify the movers and shakers in your community—those people who lead, have influence, and get things done. Read the local newspaper to find out who they are. Ask around. Watch. Follow their progress, or lack thereof. Discern and evaluate whether these influencers are doing good. Maybe, over time, you can become a mover and shaker too. That's what making a difference is all about.

Get involved and be influential.

Begin to get involved as you strategize and choose, to add your input and just good ole sweat and contributions to good efforts in the area. Join strategically, after considering the organization or involvement versus your available time and resources. Don't get "cul-de-saced" in your involvements, wasting time in places you really don't need to be. You'll be surprised how time adds up. Previously, I've joined organizations and groups that later I had to un-join due to changes or incompatibility with my goals or available time. Sometimes you just have to make a decision. Time is precious. Do the best thing, always.

It takes time to influence people and processes. You have to invest time and resources. At first it can be frustrating, because you realize you don't immediately have influence. Most of us want a drive-through window for influence, like everything else. There may be some experiences where you get to come in and quickly have influence, but usually some other experience leads to that being possible, such as when you are selected by others to influence a particular effort. But most commonly, influence is a long game. Play it that way.

There's a time to speak and a time to not speak. I believe in hanging back and gaining perspective and acceptance before barging in. I've learned to consider and weigh my words. I've also learned to regret walking away and not speaking up when I should. Sometimes you influence just by your tone, attitude, kindness, character, and ethics. I've come to appreciate the influencers who are most thoughtful, who are not a "bull in a china shop."

Perhaps more than ever I'm aware of the need to make circles bigger. Circles of influence and circles of acceptance need to get bigger. People in power need to consider those without power. We need to "be on the right side of history." For decades I've sat in the midst of people who held power, but who thought small and cold and selfishly. I do not want to leave this earth and be one of them. I want to be able to look back and be proud of myself deep within my heart and before my God. Considerations such as these fuel my head and my heart.

Invest your gifts and abilities to meet needs.

Ever utter in frustration, "Why doesn't somebody do something?" Now, go ask that question in the mirror. So, now, you must at least do something. Do you want things to improve in your area or even your country? Do something. Don't just sit and mutter and wait for everybody else.

I often read about suburban sprawl. I've lived suburban sprawl. The town and community I grew up in north of Atlanta got consumed years ago by it. I've lived in Georgia all but five years of my life, now for 25 years south of Atlanta in yet more suburbia. For more than a decade I've inserted myself into area and even regional planning meetings. I've worked to at least give a little influence in what goes where and what doesn't. I haven't fixed it all, but I've at least done something. I've been able to accomplish some things, and that's satisfying—and I'll keep chipping away at it as long and as often as I can.

We all have gifts and abilities that can benefit our community. No matter your age, background, or occupation, you can help your community. Take care of yourself as you take care of your community. Your age right now brings with it a certain perspective that would offer input needed by your community. You don't have to be a politician or urban planner or developer, but all that you've done and experienced so far can make a contribution to your community. Your occupation brings certain skills and perspectives needed by your community. Go, get involved.

The current times are full of needs that demand your investment. The things we put in concrete sometimes work for centuries. Some are a real flop, miserable failures, things that should have never been built. Some things seemed good at the time but later came to be detriments. Investing in area needs takes care of our interests by making things stronger. It's never about immediate gratification nor just about us and our needs, but "for the greater good." That's the spirit of things when we've done our best as Americans. Small, shortsighted, selfish thinking brings exactly the opposite of those high-minded ideals we've always celebrated.

When you invest, you gain. I've been voting regularly since I was 18 years old. I've always followed issues and personalities as thoroughly as possible. I've done more than my share of listening to and even engaging in conversations regarding political decisions and voting opportunities. Though I've heard many others describe their voting choices based on what it does for them, my heart and head have never allowed me to settle for that. I've always voted for the "greater good," even if it doesn't immediately benefit me, even if it goes against what you may advocate. That same attitude should fuel our investments of money, time, interest, involvement, and more in our community. Over time, over the long haul, we all benefit.

Pay attention to the "forgettables."

I love people. I'm not quite sure why, but I'm convinced much of it comes from "a fountain within," and that's the way it's supposed to be. I've wanted to sort out to whom I pay too much attention and those to whom I should pay more attention. I want to focus my attention, time, and resources on those who are deserving. To do that, it helps to learn as soon as possible whom to overlook, move on from, pass by, and yes forget. Following is my list. It's not exhaustive—even if those on it are!

- Busy bodies and troublemakers come in all shapes, sizes, and colors. They volunteer to do this. For a host of reasons, they go around finding ways to mess up people's days. They wonder out loud all the time why life is so difficult. They don't realize the problem lies largely in how they come at life. Busy bodies have to stick their nose in everybody's business. They think that by correcting and controlling others they can make things work the way they want. They live miserable lives. Troublemakers are similar in that, while picking on everybody else, they feel better about their own mess. A key to handling them is to decide early on that you're not going to take on their misery or let them scare you. You may even have to call their bluff.

- The impossibly unhappy are present in business, family, and organizational life. Many of us deal with these folks by catering to their misery and allowing them to hold us hostage so they can get their way. As examples, rearranging the seating at gatherings and feeding them what they demand come to my mind. Over time I've gained the fortitude and perspective to quietly oppose all this "rearranging" and "catering." I've learned how to sometimes quietly and sometimes confrontationally rebuff the impossibly unhappy. I've learned to "sell" this idea to everybody else involved to keep them from being unhappy while making the impossibly unhappy ones happy. Part of the art of rebuffing the impossibly happy is by reaching an arm of inclusion simultaneously—unless it's just simply someone who must go away.

- Selfish hoarders want everybody's stuff, and they want it now. Various insecurities drive them, but driven they are indeed. They think they're good people, but they'll climb right over you to get what they want. Selfish hoarders prove insatiable.

- Drama queens can be men as well as women—and I've met my share of them. They have different styles, but it all comes down to drama, drama, drama. You have to expect drama queens to emerge, no matter what you're doing or where, but don't cater to them. Give them what you can legitimately give when it's right, but hold the line when it's wrong. Be steady in dealing with drama queens; don't let them set the agenda.

None of these "forgettables" ever seem to realize they're the problem. Could you be one of them? Hard question.

Pay attention to the "unforgettables."
There are some people who need our attention the most. Sure, we need to pay attention to those we love and to those we work for. Hopefully they're among these, but here are some other groups:

- Shining stars inspire us. They give us something to look up to, something to aspire to in life. They may inspire us in faith, business, giving, understanding, fitness, sports, music, or in how to live. Learn from these shining stars. Set your sights high. Strive for your best.

- People who bless us are many. Hopefully, you can point to your parents and immediate family as your first earthly source of blessing. These are the ones who at some point knelt over you and gave you their very best in your best interest. From there, the list can grow long and deep. Savor these folks and the moments spent with them. Emulate those things they've taught you in word and deed. In turn, seek to be a blessing to everybody you encounter and in everything you say and do.

- Underdogs have to work hard to rise to the top—and we've all been the underdog at some point. If you believe in treating others as you want to be treated, be good to underdogs. If you've risen to the top, do the right thing and "send the elevator back down." No one is self-made; no one can take all the credit. Everybody gets help, gets a break, gets a leg up from somebody. "Hand outs" only last till supper time, but "help outs" can last a lifetime. When we help somebody and they make good on it, we all are better off. Think about these things the next time you have an opportunity to make a difference in an underdog's life.

Love ALL your neighbors.

We all have neighbors, whether next door or on the other side of the ranch. I've always had some good neighbors, though I've had a few who weren't. I'm talking not only about the people who live next door or down the street, but also about further out than that. Let's talk about neighbors around us, and about being neighborly.

I've had some model neighbors. I think of one with whom we enjoyed years of hearty greetings and waves across the yard. I remember the unexpected hug he gave me when I shared some bad news I had received. I think of the neighbors who've welcomed my daughter and son-in-law to their home, who look after them, who invite them into their home, who took them to the symphony. I want to be a model neighbor. It's something to aspire to be. I want to be welcoming to those around me. I want to give them a hand where I can. I want to have friendly chats in the driveway.

Some neighbors bring warm teacakes. I grew up across the road from some wonderful neighbors. In my rural neighborhood we were a little spread out, but the Stephens were all we could want for neighbors. A kind elderly couple, I went to school with their granddaughter who lived around the corner. Mr. Stephens was a longtime carpenter and had a humble workshop that I loved to visit. He built the bookshelves and cabinetry in the home where I grew up and also built hundreds of doghouses for the Marietta Sears store and thousands of other creations. Mrs. Stephens would sometimes call my mother and ask if I would go down to the road and meet her. She'd have a bread bag full of warm teacakes or angel biscuits that would melt in my mouth. The Stephens warmed my heart any time I saw them. I never heard them utter a negative word about anybody, and I certainly only heard people say good things about them. What do you give your neighbors? What do they say about you?

Most of us have some "hard to know" neighbors, especially in these days when we're more disconnected and distanced than ever. Their garage doors go up and then quickly go down. Some people want it that way. They say they just want to be left alone. They may be angry or scared or depressed. Still others go in and out their doors every day and just wish they had a nice friendly neighbor. Maybe they just haven't met you yet.

There are probably some underdogs who don't live far from you. Even if you live in an upscale neighborhood, within minutes from you there are underdogs needing a good neighbor. Maybe it's time to reach out to them.

Be a good neighbor.

There are good and bad neighbors: Which kind are you? It's great to look out the window and see the neighbors come and go, and ease out and be neighborly. Mr. Rogers made iconic fame with his song, "Won't You Be My Neighbor?" How do you answer that?

Some of your neighbors may be scary or creepy or mean or worse. It may take a lot of time to get to know them. So, what can you do? Get out more!

I've always been an outside person, so at home I'm out in my yard almost daily, at least a few minutes. Both my next-door neighbors are the same way. After that, it falls off precipitously. If you're middle-aged like me, maybe invite your younger neighbors over and get to know them or give them gardening tips or pick at their cute children. Or, mow your neighbors' yard—for them, and for you! Go for walks. Go for bike rides through and beyond your immediate neighborhood. Stop and chat with people. Share tomatoes, mutual experiences, what you have in common. Build ties. Share your waterhose, ladder, or wheelbarrow.

It's been said that fences make good neighbors. I've had neighbors where we didn't need a fence between us. I've also had neighbors where a fence or hedge helped out. At one time the neighbors behind us had quite a "collection" of stuff out back. Maybe I'd been giving them the "stink eye" and hadn't realized, but suddenly one day I found out they were going to build a privacy fence between our home and theirs, but not across the back of their property. Our neighbor next door realized what was transpiring and went to our mutual neighbor and offered to pitch in to complete the fence on their side, saying,

"I don't want to see your (stuff)." Things did improve until the neighbors behind us moved out of state but kept the home as a rental.

The first couple of renters were just fine, but then the "party crowd" moved in. These were 30-somethings who could party literally all night long, with sometimes quite a crowd. Apparently, I became the designated spokesman for the neighborhood, having to go over at 2:30 in the morning and nicely but firmly ask them to quiet down. Honestly, we all were too patient and put up with way too many nights without much sleep. I'd handle it more firmly now. Finally, they moved out. The home has now sold twice, and we're glad to have nice neighbors.

In more than 15 years of working in real estate in 15 Georgia counties, I've seen many different communities. I've also studied the dynamics of communities and towns, what makes them "livable" or not, what makes them thrive or decline. When it comes to homes, two architectural features send messages to neighbors: porches and garage doors.

I love porches! I always have. I wish our porch was much bigger, but it'll do. Many homes in our town were built without porches. They just have a front stoop. That's OK, but I love porches much better—big, shady, welcoming, inviting porches. They were originally built as an extension of the home and as a place to greet and welcome and even entertain neighbors and guests. Before air conditioning, quite often they were much more comfortable than inside on hot Summer days. Porches say to you and to all comers, "Welcome to our home." I've enjoyed many good conversations and beautiful sunsets on porches…. Then, there are garages.

Garage doors provide security that carports don't have. Unfortunately, over time, how we use garages has changed in some bad ways. More and more, it's obvious that garages have become everybody's warehouse for all the stuff they didn't used to have. Then they rent mini warehouses for still more stuff. Cars get parked in the driveway. At homes where the residents still use garages for cars, the garage has become the front door. The garage doors go up, and the garage doors go down. The homeowners are surprised when anyone arrives at their front door. They haven't even opened it in a while. These are signs of change for many people. It's evidence of the disconnect I've mentioned before and that is being talked about quite a bit these days.

So, I say let's build more porches. Let's get to know our neighbors. Let's get more connected. Let's have stronger neighborhoods and communities. I'm happy to see more places that are revitalizing by building community on the elements of connectivity, livability, walkability, bike-friendly, nature, and yes, with big, inviting porches.

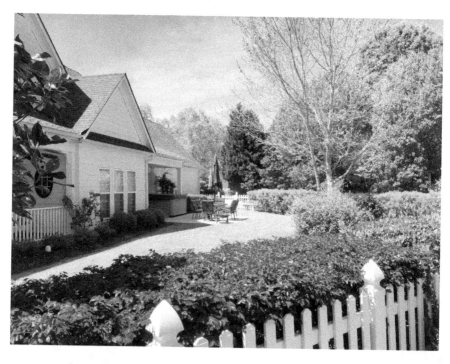

Be free of the burden of accumulation and consumerism.
Beware conspicuous consumption.

Chapter 5

Take Care of Your Things

Nowadays, it starts even before you're born. You've got stuff. In some cases, your parents don't even know where they'll put it all. Then when you're born you get more stuff. Soon, you start being told to put away all your stuff. What's a kid to do?

Look at how times have changed, even in the last 50 years or so. The proliferation of stuff in our lives is notable, while it has snuck up on most of us unaware. And, many of us are even willfully addicted to it. Study the civilizations in history, then show me any that had or have more stuff than we do now. People buy stuff to put stuff in. People go shopping and call it "retail therapy." Stuff, stuff, stuff, stuff, stuff . . .

The effects of the "big box" world on our society are well documented, though it seems many of us missed that article. Maybe we've passed the peak of the big box domination, but the effects of the shopping addiction will linger indefinitely. I remember well how different it was in my childhood.

Almost nobody had as much stuff as average folks these days. People could park their cars in their garages, even though the average home was much smaller than now. Just look around in your home, or maybe in that of your friends or neighbors. Stuff! How much of that would anybody want to pass on to their children and grandchildren? Heirloom quality? I doubt it!

I've met people who never threw anything away. They were usually rural folks who had a barn or outbuilding where they kept things because they "might need it someday." They often could repurpose or borrow parts to fabricate or repair items. They had learned this type of thing in response to what they went through during the Great Depression. They remembered what it was like to not be able to obtain things, even if they had the money. They had to be resourceful, and that meant keeping whatever resources they had, so, therefore, "resource full." But for a lot of folks who came from that era (my parents' generation), there's another ingredient.

In subsequent decades, depression-era folks made a lot of money their folks never had. Combine that with their need to "squirrel away" stuff and the advent of "shopping, shopping, shopping everywhere," a lot of basements filled up—after the closets exploded. Still others, much younger, struggling and never getting above water financially, resorted to buying whatever was "cheap" and then hoarding it to make them feel better. Again, retail therapy, they would say. And today, still others buy, buy, buy because they are bored and use "recreational shopping" as their adventures, their pastime.

Be alert to "stuff."

Stuff and the accumulating of stuff sneak up on you. You get out of college, get your own place, own just a table and chairs and an old sofa from your grandma and a bed—pretty austere. You get settled in a job, and next thing you know you fall into the modern American pattern of bringing more and more stuff home every week. It stacks up, literally.

Over a 15-year real estate career, I've dealt with client after client for whom a big factor in their home is storage of all that stuff. And they don't speak happily about it. It becomes a load to carry, a burden to bear. Some ask if we haven't touched it in a year or two, do we really need it? Also, many clients in real estate cannot finance what they desire due to the fact that they have stacked up a host of credit cards full of big box expenditures they cannot pay and that have stacked up in the house they're stuck with.

It's a little-known tenet of my Christian faith, from the teachings and life of Jesus, to practice minimalism. Jesus was homeless, contrary to what the average American in church on Sunday would tell you. Jesus had few possessions, and advocated traveling lightly: "Take nothing for the journey." Surely you would benefit from a careful, attentive reading through Scriptures focusing on this (surprising) teaching.

I have it on high authority that we should travel lightly through life. Practically, spiritually, mentally, emotionally, and psychologically—minimalism is freeing and enabling, the opposite of American consumerism and conspicuous consumption. It involves being thoughtful about how we live and about the choices we can and should make. It concerns gaining the courage to at times be different and go against the grain, and, yes, at times turning down things from family and friends.

When my children were born, I "guarded the door." I forbade anyone from buying our babies those big plastic play sets and vehicles and so forth.

Our daughters grew up (and have become well-rounded good citizens in their late 20s/early 30s) with us only letting one handheld gaming device slip through our guard. And they joined our fairly tall family in reliable, fuel-efficient cars instead of the typical gas-guzzling behemoths. They learned the joy of vacations in beautiful natural places, without having to be wowed by some manufactured spectacle. They learned the joy of close family times week in and week out that involved just simple fun and memorable moments together. They learned values as we walked through life together every day and as we reflected together on things we heard and saw and encountered.

There's a way of life and a way of looking at life that minimalism is all about. If we all had less stuff, there would be more room for beauty in our lives and in our world.

Beware of "disposable income."

Is disposable income really disposable? Even if you have money you can throw away, is that the thing to do? The term disposable income can be deceiving. It means money you have after taxes that you can spend or save as you choose. Surely you'll save it all. Of course not. There are things to buy, new technology you must have, activities your kids must participate in or they'll be disadvantaged, all those new styles of clothes constantly coming out, exciting new cars and trucks and SUVs, and those exotic trips you need to be taking.

Can you really throw away your extra income? Is it burning a hole in your pocket? Maybe you should just toss it out the window. Disposable income is a bad concept. Most of us agree, but then go out week in and week out and spend money we really don't have on all sorts of stuff that in the long run makes no appreciable sense. Poof! It's gone. Easy come, easy go.

Most of us work hard for our money. We rush and make long stressful commutes to a job that also may be long and stressful, and then do it all over again and again. The money we make may be hard won, but especially these days it can go away easily. Many of the things we buy, much of our economy, and our very attitude about those things are too much about being disposable—throwaway society, we call it. We need to awaken ourselves to the fact that most of us have developed a disposable mentality. For everything from straws to relationships, they're all disposable, and that affects our perspectives. With a disposable mentality, the value of things changes: it cheapens everything. Is anything precious?

Currently, there is a controversy over straws. Actually, plastic straws are not one of the most critical issues we face, but what folks don't realize is how many million straws get used daily worldwide, and how that impacts wildlife, waterways, and people. Straws are just one part of a huge problem with plastics and their disposal and even their manufacturing.

We need to make changes in what we use and how we use it. It's not only what we do but also our attitudes about it that matter. In similar fashion, in personal relationships, in the workplace, in business dealings, and yes in politics, the disposable mentality is a huge factor.

Know the value and cost of things.

I learned early what things really cost. I saw firsthand what a fascination with "more and cheaper" did to individuals and to us collectively. I saw what happened to the look of the land as we forsook Main Street for Big Box. I saw the price of cheap versus craftsmanship. I saw the resultant multilevel societal problems of this modern-day gold rush for "more, cheaper, now." I'm starting to see us try to fix all that. I am hopeful it continues. We need to develop a mindset and an eye for quality.

Long ago I learned that I'd rather have fewer but higher quality things. I began to eschew anything associated with a disposable mentality. I learned to be frugal and to do without instead of wasting money on things that "go to pot." I hate "saving money" in decisions that end up costing more money. What often gets sold as being "conservative" is not really less expensive over time. Some things that "save money" actually cost more in the long run, especially when you have to fix them. That doesn't appeal to me.

When I graduated from college and a week later my wife and I were married, I quickly learned some things about spending my own money. What is "cheaper" often is not cheaper. I hate spending money three times when I could have paid a little more the first time to have it done right. As time has gone on, I've become more insistent on that. I've also learned deeply the value of people, nature, truth, and other intangibles. What do you deeply value?

Purchase "indisposables" instead of "disposables."

Stop a minute and look at how much stuff you throw out at home and at work. Is all that really necessary? Years ago, I began to become aware of the huge amount of disposables in our lives. It was pointed out to me that not only is this a practical concern, but also an ethical and even a spiritual concern. Increasingly over the years, I make my purchasing decisions to include more about where products come from, what's in them, and how we will dispose and/or recycle them.

I've never liked cheap or trendy clothes. I'd rather have a couple of new, classic-styled shirts of good quality that will be around several years than 10 new, cheap, trendy shirts or other items that will fall apart before the year is over. I've felt the same about other purchases, for example, the cheap furniture my wife and I bought early on that fell apart too quickly. I love our now-18-year-old lawnmower that cranks on the first pull and runs great; it's so much better than the several cheaply made mowers we had prior to that. When the affordability question gets posed to me on things like this, I always counsel the inquirer to look at a series of expenditures he or she will admit to. Usually and quickly, I can round up the extra cash needed in that person's budget to buy the better item.

It's not just because I'm now north of 55 years old, but because this is where I'm at. As much as I can, I buy things that aren't disposable. I look for products that are biodegradable, recyclable, or lasting. Sure, I can't get everything to fall in those categories, but why shouldn't I want to achieve this? If they're not biodegradable or recyclable, then hopefully they're items I can keep forever or pass on to others. It's a mentality—perhaps an "heirloom" mentality—to develop or a way to minimize my impact on the environment.

I sometimes joke about how my wife and I are into long-term relationships, such as our marriage and many of our possessions. We've been married for more than 35 years, since age 21. We've been in our current home for 15 years. And, between us and our daughters, we've had nine cars, four of which are still with us and running great. While we sometimes buy new clothes, I know I've got outfits I've had as long as 15 years. I'm into things I want to keep around. I try to make sure of that before I obtain them.

Whether it's clothes or cars or relationships, I choose wisely. I look for dependability as a top criterion. I don't care how good it looks or how fast it goes. If it's full of drama or breaking down all the time, it's not desirable. Another criterion is sustainability and minimalism. It matters how things are made and how things last. Both affect where things go. Whether it's clothes or cars or relationships, I like things that age well, that are timeless in their beauty, that I'm glad to have around year after year and decade after decade. Think about these criteria with everything and everyone you have in your life.

Consider the overall costs of your home.

Home sweet home: it's where you land each night. It's where they're supposed to let you in every time you come to the door. Hopefully, it's a welcoming place. Let's look at taking care of yourself by taking care of your home.

Home is something many of us take for granted. Most of us grow up in a home that is provided for us. We proceed through however many years of school, then are faced with the question of where to live and how to pay for it. Our home is the most expensive purchase we'll make, followed by cars and health care expenses.

During my 15 years in real estate of helping clients, I took seriously what I did every day in helping people deal with their most precious and most expensive possession. It's more than money and square footage and carpet. For me, it's more than just another sale. It's personal. It's where memories are made. It's where people celebrate and where they worry.

Buying and owning a home can have many expensive ramifications. Most folks don't know what they don't know. They need someone with their best interests in mind and at heart.

Americans live in homes of many shapes and sizes. Currently, most of us live in homes that are approximately twice as large as those in 1960. What we consider essential in a home has evolved and continues to evolve. If you're in the market for a home, what is best for you? Beyond the particulars of the city or town, let's explore some things about home that really matter.

Aside from being in what we think is a pretty place with pretty surroundings, our homes should be affordable, maintainable, sustainable, and livable. We take care of ourselves when we choose a home that meets these criteria.

• Your home should be one that you can afford to pay for, heat and cool, and maintain both now and in the future. Unless you're independently and infinitely wealthy, I would suggest consulting with a financial advisor. This consultation, which in some cases may take only minutes, can help you keep perspective about the biggest transaction you'll ever make.

Next, unless you have the money in bank accounts to stroke a check, get preapproval from a quality lender. If you have an excellent real estate agent, he or she can connect you with top local lenders. This gives you two things you need: preapproval in hand that helps you in negotiating for the home you want (a necessary prerequisite) and confirmation for what you can afford. (Of course, you shouldn't spend up to the limit of what you can get preapproved for! Don't be "house poor.")

- Now, you might be ready to find and negotiate for the home you want. After affordability, there's the question of maintainability. The way homes are built, even architecture and "accessories," can pose huge questions regarding maintenance. That half-acre of deck: It's good now, but what will it cost to repair and/or replace in the future? Do you really want to be a pool owner? And what about that worn-out HVAC unit, the roof, the septic system, and the drainage problem, and on and on? What will a home warranty cover? What about the neighboring properties and their effect on the value of yours? There's much to consider.

- Okay, so you're just trying to afford and purchase a home. Who has time to consider sustainability? Our impact on the earth is great and, collectively, is not sustainable. Many of us are making efforts to have less impact. One of the biggest decisions is to limit our commute. Another is to have less home and to make that home as efficient as possible. Water and energy use inside and outside is key. And, yes, more of us will have energy savings from solar and wind power in coming years.

- Then, there's livability. Can you age in place in your home? At some point this will be a consideration. Make your home choice strategically and intentionally. Consider how you'll use your home and how you'll get around. Consider the community you want to be a part of, not just the home.

Choose a home based on location and maintenance needs.

Location is relative to everything around it. A mistake many homebuyers make these days is going to a website and clicking through and going "pretty house, pretty house, ugly house, ugly house, ugly house, pretty house." Then they dig further into the pretty ones and call their agent and say, "Let's go see it!" And, many agents won't slow them down even for a minute, but just blindly set up the visits and away they go.

Sure, start with pretty. But make sure behind the pretty it fits all your criteria. Sooner or later you will find out that the old adage about the best-known phrase in real estate is true: location, location, location. Location can trump everything else about your home. There are many wonderful, pretty homes in bad locations. Location matters for your enjoyment of the home in the present, and it matters for your resale value in the future.

A key component of location relates to family commutes. Thousands of buyers ignore this issue when house hunting. In metro Atlanta, for example, we average some of the longest and most stressful daily commutes on the planet. Add us all together, and metro Atlantans drive to the sun and back every day! That's more than 186 million miles. So, when people looking for homes tell me they're fine with the commute and can look in five different counties, I at least attempt to slow them down a minute and discuss commutes—the time, the gas, the pollution, the costs, the wear and tear on cars and on people, the hours of living that will be lost.

But tell me, how much is it worth getting up at 5:00 a.m. and driving maybe three hours a day, fighting it out with everybody on the road and getting home at 7:00 p.m. and doing it all over each day and being a vegetable on the weekend? The toll is tremendous in many ways. Before you commit to all these things, count the costs. Increasing numbers of people, especially millennials, are demanding a change.

Again, no matter how wonderful the home is, if there are location problems, that will negate all the other features. There are many handy resources that can help make this possible. Tops to me are the online and app mapping services. Look up 123 Smith Street, for example, and take an initial look at where the home is located versus whatever is around it. Next, look at the satellite view. Then, go see it live and in person.

There's "macro location" and "micro location"—both of which matter, especially over the long term. Macro location is where the home is versus commute locations and other criteria considered important. Micro location is the position on that very street.

This brings up the issue of why the last lots to go in a neighborhood are often the worst lots. Maybe they sit in a hole or back up to major power lines or a railroad track or a noisy highway or have other undesirable factors. I've seen buyer after buyer go for the pretty house hanging off a cliff or sitting in a swamp because "it's new construction" or "it has all new appliances" or "they'll pay $10,000 in closing costs." (Real estate appraisers see the same thing all the time: not everything is awesome.) I told all my real estate clients about my "So I can sleep at night policy." In other words, whether they were buyers or sellers or both, I always told them about any pitfalls related to a property. Then, it was up to the clients as to what they wanted to do.

When I talk about location versus "where you live," I mean giving further thought to where you do most of your activities, including at work and when not at work. Jot down the things you do regularly, such as grocery shopping, recreational activities, church and civic involvement, and more. Note the distance of each activity from your home or intended home, plus the commute time. Let this help guide your decisions about where to live and the involvements. Count the costs. You'll be glad you did.

In addition to determining the best location and other factors related to choosing a home, think about maintenance. This is where home and other inspectors can be invaluable. Keep in mind that, especially in the Southeast, water is perhaps enemy number one for your home. Roofs are a primary big-ticket item. They're the first line of defense against water! At the bottom, holding it all up is the foundation, critical to support and, again, one of the places most attacked by water. The heat and air system can be a big concern and expense. And, the plumbing and sewer/septic system, while unpleasant to deal with and even more expensive, all matter greatly. Then there are other considerations: floor joists, termites, siding, electrical boxes, windows—all part of the picture of home sweet home. The more sturdy and low maintenance and high quality these and all other components are, the less expense and headaches you'll have. Take care of yourself by taking care of your home.

Examine the "real" costs of your vehicle.

Sometimes it seems I've spent half my life driving. It's the American way. When you look at our collective love for all things related to cars and trucks, even the music around it all, you must realize how huge a thing driving is for us.

I love to drive; I always have. I love going places, seeing things, and I love everything about driving a vehicle. I even drove big buses for 15 years for my college, a school system, and churches—thousands of miles, across seven states, without a scratch. I've been able to, so far, drive all these years without an accident and to do it smoothly and calmly. To get from point A to B that is not served by alternative forms of transportation, here we go in the car.

We don't realize the actual costs of cars and getting around. I always remind people who argue that alternative transportation and mass transportation require subsidizing that they've never driven on a road that wasn't subsidized. We need to face these facts and have legitimate, truthful conversations about the challenges facing our society. Even if we got all the cars solar-powered tomorrow—and even if they sounded and performed like powerful V8s—we'd still have a logistical problem, especially the way our infrastructure is set up currently.

We're not good at moving traffic, and we're not good at reducing traffic. All those solar-powered cars—which could free us from carbon-based fuels and the problems they cause—would still face the problem of too many in the same place at the same time. And of course, somebody would find a way to have an accident and clog things up worse. Also, there's the usually overlooked costs of the time we lose stuck at traffic lights and the commute itself—and the stress and strain of fighting traffic that most of us are resigned to thinking it just has to be that way. It's why some of us have been working for years to bring change to all of this. Meanwhile, we drive.

I started pumping gas at my dad's store in the early 70s. On that corner I saw all kinds of cars and trucks and people driving them. Years later I spent most of a decade in a dealership service department, the oldest of its brand in metro Atlanta. I've been around cars a lot. I've studied the automotive press for years. I know the importance of genuinely good cars, and I've studiously kept up with which ones make the grade. My advice is to purchase a truly good car—one for which there's little fuss, aggravation, and expense—and then take impeccable care of it. There are all sorts of cars that go fast and handle well and look great, but to do that and to be reliable and fuel-efficient and last a long time, that's where my money will go. Take care of yourself as you take care of a good car.

I cannot say enough about the importance of good gas mileage. Thankfully and increasingly, automakers are converting their fleets to hybrid and electric cars. Meanwhile, especially in the South, monster trucks and huge SUVs rule the day. My first car was a 1969 Chevy pickup, but it was a different day and we used it with our farming and our store. Most of us cannot justify, from a financial or environmental perspective, something that gets 15 miles per gallon on the highway. And, if ethics and science matter, then these perspectives matter. Take care of yourself as you take care of our environment and your pocketbook by insisting on good miles per gallon.

Take care of your vehicle.

Maybe it was because I grew up pumping gas and checking oil at my dad's store. Maybe it was my own young intuition. Maybe it was because of my first new car that I only had for just over a year. That car about drove me to drink. There was an unbelievable list of things that went wrong the first year. All those things and more taught me to choose better, to do my homework, and to take care of my car. I've never been a mechanic. I own a small assemblage of tools, but folks have rarely found me tooling under the hood of a car. But I can tell you a thing or two about taking care of your car and why.

In my dad's store, I grew up listening to people talk about everything under the sun. I pondered those things I heard, tested out some, and came to my own conclusions over time. Cars and servicing cars were among the many categories of conversation. Then, time ticked quickly by, I was married, and we were on our own. My money was my money, and I had to manage it. Quickly, I determined that for factory service and parts and training, I couldn't beat the dealership. For a number of years, I was the customer. Then, a turn of events led to me working at a dealership and eventually becoming assistant manager of the service department.

For most of a decade I helped deliver the best possible service to thousands of people. More than half the cars we touched every day had 150,000 miles on them. During the time I was there, we set the highest customer satisfaction index scores and achieved our make's award for number one in America for

"Fix It Right the First Time" scores. Getting it right every day meant everything to me, and I still have former clients reach out to me.

I'm a customer again, but I still want it "right every time." I have high expectations. And, yes, I know my way around in "that world." Remember what I recounted earlier about having only nine cars in 35 years of marriage, including with our two daughters, and that four of those cars are still with us? I point to quality cars, well chosen, with consistent care over time.

A vehicle has two pedals that are very important: the gas and brakes. I have spent more than my share of miles behind the wheel, including all those years driving buses. Once, I was swapping some stories with a truck-driving friend, and he told me a little gem about "those two pedals." Treat them both lightly, he said. Whichever one you're pressing, especially pressing hard, you're costing money. You're either burning gas or you're burning brakes. The easier and smoother you can go on both, the easier you are on money (and resources).

Since I was 15 and with a learner's license, I've always worked at operating a vehicle smoothly in addition to safely. Smooth is good. Safe is tops. Part of safe is smooth. Learn about it. Take care of yourself and others by the way you drive.

Basic maintenance, including that of tires, is primary. I've always been amazed at the worn-out stuff people drive—around my daughters and now my grandchildren. I remember many times at the dealership when I had to tell customers, "I can see the air in your tires they're so worn out." These were slick tires with the cords showing, making them unsafe and illegal. I see the same thing all the time as I walk through parking lots. Your tires are your most important connection to the road. Maintain them. Keep them properly inflated, rotated, balanced, and aligned. Don't just go, go, go. Stop and check your tires. Lives are on the line. Good maintenance saves lives, but it also saves time and money.

Here's another thing I've told people hundreds of times: It's more important to stop than it is to go. As much as we want and need our cars to go, it's even more important to make them stop when needed. The first thing with managing speed is how to control it and how to stop it. So, nothing is more important on our cars than the brakes. It's important that the brakes are maintained and working, and it's important that we use them properly.

Most people stop too late. Most use the brakes too much due to the fact that they are traveling too closely to other cars. Most people don't stop smoothly. Many people have an apparent "conveyor belt mentality" when driving that propels them onward when, in fact, they should be braking and slowing down and avoiding a hazard that is stacking up in front of them. We do not drive on a conveyor belt, and we can and should be cognizant and respond proactively rather than too late.

People get lucky in traffic amazingly often. They also get unlucky, and the results can be expensive and often tragic. Take care of yourself and others as you drive. It's serious business out there.

Car maintenance also involves the outward appearance. You may never own a bottle of wax or wash your car yourself, but regularly keep it washed and waxed. It's partly a point of pride, but it's also part of maintaining what is your second-most expensive possession next to your home (unless you have your priorities really right and your bike is worth more than your car). So, if you won't do it yourself, have a detailer wash and wax your vehicle regularly. It will protect your investment for the long term. (I've always said it makes cars drive better, too.)

Many things attack our paint finishes, especially acid rain (pollution in the rain), tree sap, bugs, and bird droppings. Get them off quickly and regularly! Drive-through car washes don't get all that stuff off. And, don't use your car's windshield washer either. That solution is hard on the clearcoat finish.

For several years now, I've cleaned my cars' exteriors at local self-service car washes. I first check for grit in the brushes, then proceed to wash the vehicles, finishing with the clearcoat protector and wax applications. Self-service car washes are quicker and more convenient than at home and actually save water—especially the ones that recycle water. Back home in my garage, as needed, I do hand-waxing and other detailing. Plus, I keep our four bicycles, our golf cart, and my antique tractor clean and waxed. A little while in the garage with the fan making a breeze and the radio on and turning a vehicle to gleaming: it's therapeutic. Use a little elbow grease, and enjoy the satisfaction.

I also take care of my other car: my bike. People around me often hear me say much about my love for all things bikes and cycling. I long for, look for, and am working for the day when we all can make more of our trips by bike. There are countries where people already do that, and happily. No, not everything can be done by bike, but much more could be. The challenges that face us personally as a society demand better thinking than we've been giving.

We must do better. And, in the process, a lot of things could be more fun and enjoyable for everybody. I predict the bike will be one mode of transportation that we will see used much more in coming years. And, we're all going to have a lot more fun as that happens.

Let stuff mean less, and instead serve a purpose.

Most of us are too much about stuff. We need an intentional and methodical reordering of our priorities, obsessions, and even of our economy—personally and as a society.

I remember reading a disturbing book in a college sociology class titled *Entropy*, by Jeremy Rifkin and Ted Howard. It was not bedtime reading or "cheer you up" reading. It challenged us to grapple with issues that people 100 years ago did not face. It caused us to focus on the obvious fact that our runaway consumption and abuse of the world's resources are destructive to our planet and, in turn, to us. Too many of us blindly dismiss this as talk by extremists and nerds and "those people"—a socialist ploy. And, we hear politicians and other influencers who champion the bigger and better American way.

Keep the wheels of progress turning, they say. Keep turning out those American products, widening those American roads, digging up whatever we can burn to make things go. But the warning signs have been on the horizon for decades and, increasingly, the actual problems, too. Loving our country, our world, and our children just might require us to face facts and make decisions we might initially balk at or resist in the interest of long-term prosperity itself.

I've had to learn to look at my stuff differently. Even the author of my faith urged that we not be so desirous of things that "rust" and "corrode." It first means that we collect less of the tangibles and collect more of the intangibles in life. The older I get and the more I learn and observe, I realize how true is that ancient yet timely wisdom.

Letting stuff mean less can result in a resetting of our life goals. I've gotten to where I can identify certain possessions that some would call the American Dream that I'd be embarrassed to have. It means so much less "keeping up with the Joneses" (or the Kardashians) or whoever it is with whom you're comparing. It means thinking a lot less about what you want to get, and even what you still do want may look so much different than what you had in mind. It may be scary at first, but oh the freedom it brings. We also need to be free of the burden of accumulation and consumerism.

I used to see "all these things" and began to buy in a little to the "pursuit of the American Dream." At some point, thankfully early enough, I realized where life could truly be found. I became more and more turned off by "conspicuous consumption" and how it all looked. Disney's movie *Wall-E* from 2008 provided a surprising modern satire or fable that captured and spoke to conspicuous consumption. If you listen closely, you can see parallels between its story and your own life. We need to make changes in our attitudes, choices, and lifestyle while there's still time.

Calculate the real cost of your purchases.

My dad used to give me a little money when I got to driving age. Well, I worked for him much of the time at his store—$20 here, $20 there. Back in the 70s, that could last me longer than you would believe. Even then, Dad would often be surprised that I still had money left over—even after I'd been on a date. (The girl was surprised, too! Okay, I was a "cheap date.") I quickly learned to watch my money. I never wanted to let it all evaporate. I realized that money could be fleeting and that I needed to manage it well.

What is it about sales that makes money burn holes in our pockets? It seems I meet more and more people who spend money they really don't have for things they really don't need because some ad or some person has gotten into their head that they must have it. Sometimes it's a little laughable. Sometimes it gets tragic and sad. One of the best ways to save money is to not spend it.

I hate spending money three times. I've always been drawn to quality. I learned early the hard way that cheaper isn't always better, and more often than not it isn't. Whether it comes to clothes or car service or a new bike or whatever, I'd rather do my homework and pay a little more for lasting quality than to get it cheap and have to pay three times to get it right.

Countless times in our service department years ago, we'd be called upon to fix a car that had "already been fixed." When we diagnosed and prescribed a fix and gave an updated estimate, quite often the client would reply, "But Bubba's Garage was so much cheaper." My reply, prefaced politely, was "Well, our factory-trained technicians have diagnosed the problem. The actual cost of Bubba's repair will be what he has already charged you plus what we are charging to fix it correctly." It's cheaper to pay more to get it right the first time instead of investing in flimsy, cheap, shoddy, unreliable products and services.

Another thing that comes up all the time is why I prefer to buy from local businesses and eat at local restaurants as opposed to the big boxes and chain restaurants. I'd rather pay a little more if I have to and to support my local economy than support "bigger and cheaper." I prefer to get one or two quality items rather than six of them that are cheap, trendy, and poorly made—with the buttons popping off in a month.

A little forethought and consideration can help us make the best decisions with our money. I've witnessed and heard for at least 40 years about "being conservative" and about "saving money" and a host of other bits of wisdom and myth. I've watched where many of those choices led us, and again and again I found them shortsighted and ultimately more expensive.

I look at transportation projects that were shortsighted and "saved money" but that are now proving more costly: we are having to pay many times over to attempt to retrofit and fix what we knew way back when should have been done better. Yes, I'm talking about those old "widen the roads" and "we don't want it here" transportation votes that are now costing us immeasurably. Oh, and there's the "let's run three major interstates right through the middle of downtown" syndrome that's driving us all nuts and the costs of which will never be counted fully, with ramifications on so many levels. Take it up a level higher and look at the untold costs of ongoing environmental degradation that we're already paying and will be paying much more in the future. I always point out that it's the bottom line we should be looking at—not that "false bottom" line that so often gets used.

Save money by doing without and making smarter choices.

I jokingly apologize every so often to my wife for things I haven't gotten her. I'll see a commercial for indulgent jewelry and apologize that I've never bought her some. Various sights bring out this joke every so often. I also apologize to her that I haven't been a tremendous "provider" for her and our daughters. About this time, she starts getting nauseated and tells me to stop it!

All this joking and some sarcasm mixed in aside, we've been clear for all of our married years with our values and wishes. One of the secrets for our happiness and even success comes from just not wanting as much as everybody else. We've realized thousands of times that there are many things we just don't need. In the process, we've saved so much money by just doing without. But I keep on apologizing!

While I may not want or have as much as some people, I've learned to make smart choices in my purchases. I like decisiveness, but I like it better after I've done my homework. I like that in leaders, too. I don't shoot from the hip unless I know what I'm doing. After some mistakes early on that "bit me," I learned to do my research before deciding, before purchasing, before committing. And, I like to do my homework from sources that I can best determine to be objective. I want the truth; I don't want a bias. I don't like to be disappointed later on. Read. Be curious. Listen. Watch. Think. There comes a time when you should make a decision. Be prepared.

Part of making smart choices may involve spending a little more money. I try not to "grind" businesses or people in business for pennies. I have a real disdain for people who do. I first met those kinds at my dad's store. I've met them countless times in business, and continue to meet them in my business these days. I've met even more folks who think they're brilliant if they make a fortune off of folks, but obviously resent anyone who might make a dollar off of them. I've never had much time for these folks. They're also the kinds of folks who've "done well" but who whine and gripe all the time about all the "hoards" of people who want handouts, yet manipulate the system so they don't have to pay their fair share. Over the years I've proved myself as a loyal customer. I'll hang in there with you if I feel you're deserving. I'll also pay a little more for local or sustainable products.

Recently, it came up again. We were in a small town we know well, and a decision was being made about where to shop for certain items. We were urged to go to the "big box." We made clear we were going local and smaller. We paid only a few more dollars at the locally owned business, and from what we've studied about "strong towns" and from what we've observed, we made the right decision. We do this all the time—where we eat, what we eat, and where we get our fruits and vegetables and other things. Study the local and sustainable movements. Learn where things come from and how they get there, and start to grasp the big picture. It'll make you change your ways.

Plan for the future.

I'm no financial expert, but regarding saving money for retirement and health, if I had it to do all over again, I would have started earlier and invested more. But we're working hard at it in this stage of life. It is a help to have the opportunity. It is in all our best interests to save, save, save. Reality is that circumstances are unpredictable at any stage of life and quite often they're not ideal. Again, this is a prime reason to stay out of debt as much as possible and to save, save, save. It's no secret that Americans these days are on average woefully underprepared for retirement, and coming decades could see many crises caused by this situation. Here are some prime causes:

• Many people do not think past today. Or, if they do, they keep telling themselves, "We'll save for retirement tomorrow." They keep putting it off. Their money continually gets spent on something else—something more immediate, something tangible, something that's in front of them. Tomorrow always seems so far away, until it's here.

• Ours is a modern world of instant gratification. We want it now, we expect it now, and most often within 90 seconds. Since we often don't think past the moment, we don't prepare for the future. We say, "I want that now," so we get it. If we're truthful, what we get now may not matter at all in six months. How much could that investment have grown if it had been put toward retirement or a rainy day?

• Most of us didn't see what has been termed the "Lost Decade" coming until it was here. Even then, we kept thinking that next week we would pop out of it. But the Great Recession took a lot of time, and for many people, financially, it was a lost decade. This means that many folks are essentially 10 years behind where they would be in savings if all that debacle hadn't happened. That's time and money none of us can get back.

• Many people have responded to the times we experienced by "dragging anchor" and not investing until politics looked like they wanted them to look. We all lost over that. Other people became more selfish, more protective, fearful that someone would get what they have. Again, we all lost over that. But thankfully, we recovered better and faster than some of us thought we would. But it has been an uneven recovery, and many people have been left floundering in our modern-day "junk economy" while opportunities that a new, greener economy would present remain beyond our grasp. Meanwhile, nobody is getting any younger.

- Financial disasters are as old as time, but way too many still happen these days. When the Great Recession hit—which, thankfully, did not become another depression, as it well could have—thousands of people were discovered to be one job loss away from foreclosure. Add to that the way our health care system works in what many of us believe should be the greatest nation in the world, and yet another source of financial disaster hit still more thousands. Some of them were the same people who experienced foreclosures. I sold foreclosures for two banks and the FDIC during the recession, and I hope I never have to do that again. It wasn't good for anybody. I'd rather make my money off a healthy economy that works for everybody. We'll all be better off.

All these and more are reasons you and I need to be saving more for tomorrow. Country singer Garth Brooks has a hit song titled "If Tomorrow Never Comes." Well, tomorrow does come, and we best be preparing for it today. Take care of yourself, and take care of your retirement savings today.

Rainy days come to all of us. Some of us get more sunny days than others. Some get more rainy days than others. We need to prepare for rainy days. It's always a happier situation if we're not "scraping the barrel" financially or in any other way.

To ensure future financial security, we must plan carefully. I suggest working with a trustworthy financial planner. I hired a personal friend as mine, and he is both trustworthy and competent. Root out that person in your life with whom you can develop and implement a financial plan that gets you to your retirement savings and other financial goals. Take your advisor and the plan seriously, and contribute to your plan early and often.

I would also encourage you to develop multiple sources of income. The famed "Oracle of Omaha" Warren Buffett, one of the world's richest persons, is noted for urging us all to have multiple sources of income at every stage of life. This plan may take a while to develop and may well include investments in multiple accounts. But by starting to map it out today, and working at things that are "in your wheelhouse," who knows what might develop over time for you? Take care of your finances, both for today and tomorrow.

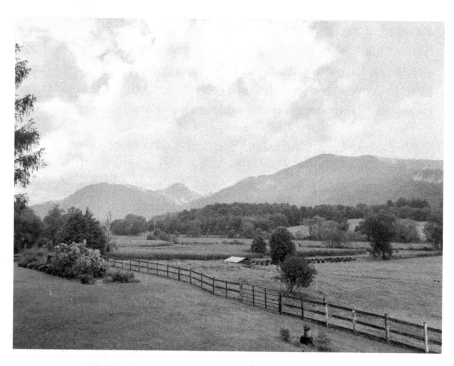

Our environment is precious. Nothing is more important for us.

Chapter 6

Take Care of Your World

For as long as I can remember, I've loved the outdoors. One of my earliest memories as a tot was being outside in my pedal car, trying to get an ID on a bird. I can see me there in the driveway by our home in Acworth, Georgia, looking up after what I believe was a cardinal.

Whenever I'm inside, I'm looking outside. (That didn't always work out in school, as I remember.) I can't say enough to encourage you to take care of yourself by taking care of your natural world and by getting out in it often.

My lifelong love has been my world, the outdoors, the natural world. I'm happiest when I'm out in nature or studying about nature. The scenery, the trees, the birds, the animals, waterfalls, mountain streams, the marshes, ocean sunsets, even a swamp in winter all have beauty.

Living my first memorable years on a Georgia horse and cattle ranch gave me many opportunities to be impressed by nature's beauty. Sure, there were new little calves and foals to delight in, but beyond that there were the pasture views and the forests. There was always something to discover and enjoy, each day and in all seasons. My love of that atmosphere has never let up.

By early elementary school, and as soon as I could read, a love of nature awakened in me and I told people that I wanted to be a wolf biologist. Unfortunately, that dream was never realized. Life took a different course, but I've kept up my studies and involvement in nature to this day—from subscribing to *Ranger Rick* magazine and watching *Wild Kingdom* with Marlin Perkins as a boy and gobbling up all sorts of nature books and magazines; to college studies in geology and geography; to continued study in climate change, biodiversity, endangered species, habitat loss, and a multitude of other subjects.

My lifelong fascination with birds and mammals continues to offer something to see, study, discover, and keep up with every day. Add to that, over the last 10 years I've been a board member of our local Southern Conservation Trust, which now protects more than 45,000 acres across Georgia and beyond. As I'm known for saying, we're protecting land "just for the rain to fall and the birds to tweet."

Consider nature as home.

The more you comprehend how critical nature is to your very being, the more precious it becomes to you. Nature is not a place to visit; nature is home. Maybe you're not at home in nature. Maybe you think nature is "icky." I would say you need to get out a lot more. You need to begin to discover the beauty and comfort of nature, while at the same time learning to know and respect those forces of nature that could harm you. Nature truly is home, and we should overcome our modern separation and alienation and detachment from it.

In *The Reaffirmation of Prayer*, theologian Glenn Hinson speaks about how our alienation from nature is indicative and symptomatic of our alienation from God. I have to agree. It's not too late for you to get out there more. Reach into nature wherever it is close to you, hopefully right out your back door. Begin or begin again to take it in. Watch it, listen to it, smell it, taste it, grasp it, study it, ponder it, enjoy it. Never again go back inside and feel like nature is strange.

Think of nature as something very familiar.

I'm continually amazed by folks who have zero interest in nature. Observing and liking nature should be like breathing. It is the very air we breathe, the source of the water we drink.

Recently I was in a very unnatural place in our town, putting items in my car in a parking lot in front of a store. The parking lot has a scattering of trees carefully placed by design to allow for maximum parking. As I loaded the car, out of one of the nearby trees came a bird's song I didn't recognize. Then I heard it again.

As has been my lifelong habit, I headed toward the singing to see the bird I was hearing. That's how I've always done it since I was a boy, and that's how I've learned to identify so many birds. I'd hear birdsong, approach the sound, see the birds, and either recognize them or note their features and go look them up in my bird books.

As I neared the tree in the parking lot, two yellow warblers flew past me. I gasped in delight, having wanted to see yellow warblers all my life and never before had this opportunity. I followed them across the parking lot to the trees they'd flown to, and out they flew again.

I couldn't help but want to discover what was making the sounds I was hearing. It started by just paying attention and being curious—nothing foreign, even in a place not conducive to nature.

Enjoy the health benefits of nature.

Folks like me who love to be out and about in nature would do it even if it didn't add to our health. We'd just be out there reveling in the beauty of it all. But study after study proves that being in nature is great for our physical, mental, and spiritual health. Being in nature relaxes you; puts things into perspective; gives you a natural workout as you hike, bike, swim, climb, or scramble wherever you go; and makes your spirit tender. Spiritually, nature helps you get more in touch with the Creator. For me, as both a person of faith and as a lifelong student of science, nature brings both together as I seek to comprehend and appreciate it all through immersion in nature.

Play in nature, no matter your age.

Three words—adults, play, nature—may seem foreign to many of us. For too many adults, play is a forgotten thing. Many of us take ourselves and life way too seriously and somberly. Play is for kids. There's money to make, things to prove, challenges to conquer, competition to beat. Play in nature? First, I've got to return to play, and now you're asking me to do it out in icky nature?

Playing in nature is exactly what many of us need. Play may come easiest as we follow our children into the woods and engage with them in whatever play arises, unplanned and unscripted as ours was long ago. Play may come as a loving couple escapes for a date in nature and finds themselves marveling and laughing and maybe kissing on a creek bank.

Over the past 35 years my wife and I have found ourselves playing in nature in a variety of ways: exploring a lake near our first home together and coming upon a beautiful red fox, driving through the night together and marveling at the beautiful lightning we were witnessing in the sky ahead, putting up bird feeders and birdhouses at every home we've occupied, witnessing hundreds of cedar waxwings eating cedar berries one snowy day, capturing a photo of me with our then-two-year-old daughter on my back and hanging onto my neck as I crept down a rock to get us to the foot of a 200-foot-tall waterfall. The stories could go on and on and still are happening as we play in nature.

Encourage children to play in nature.

Perhaps the most powerful book of our time that argues why it's so important to immerse children in nature is Richard Louv's *Last Child in the Woods*. This work explores problems that have arisen because of kids not playing outside—boredom, obesity, attention disorders, depression—and offers solutions and inspiration for getting them back out there.

I remember how I couldn't wait to get home from school and play outside my rural home every day. My mother would call me in for a bit when *Mr. Rogers* came on TV, but otherwise I would spend the afternoon playing outside in all seasons.

During the summer I'd run all over our place barefooted, sometimes imitating the barefoot running of Ron Ely in the *Tarzan* show of that day. Other times I had a pine sapling "rifle" and played Fess Parker's version of *Daniel Boone*. Of course, I always played around our cattle in the pasture and sometimes around our hogs in the hog pen. I'd climb up in "my" maple tree and while away some time, watching the robins work our yard and the blue jays in the oak trees, waiting to see a half mile down the road my dad's blue 1965 Chevy pickup coming out of the entrance to the ranch as he headed home.

What do your kids get to do?

Protect the environment.

There are many matters our society is arguing—make that screaming—about these days. Whether or not it's the hot-button issues of the moment, there are serious issues we need to handle. Human rights, racial tensions, violence, economic opportunity, and many more deserve proper attention. But stack up whatever issues you believe to be a priority, and I'll argue that the future of our environment and climate change supersede them all. If we don't get this right, all others will pale in comparison.

Climate change is not something theoretical out there in the future, but something real and powerful and happening already. Most adults I know look askance at teenagers who are always testing the limits, breaking the rules, trying to see how fast they can go around the curve, testing the laws of physics, just being plain stupid, seeing how far they can take it before hitting the wall. We adults are doing the same thing by ignoring the weight of science, decades of reports, change that has happened in our lifetime, and commonsense, and just believing what folks with an agenda want us to believe. Why do we put so much money and effort into seeing how far we can push things?

There are too many signs to ignore about the problems of climate change and fossil fuels. And, we do have alternatives, and our energy companies need to be proactive and become exactly what they should be—energy companies. I hope I live to see the day when my grandchildren ask me, "Why did you all dig up things and burn them for so long when you knew better?"

It's not just climate change, though, that is the "800-pound gorilla in the room." We've heard for years about problems with the air we breathe. Though there have been many improvements, there's still a long way to go. Water is another huge problem, and will become more so. We think water is an unlimited resource—we turn on the faucet and it comes out. Most of us don't comprehend how precious water is, where it really comes from, the "water cycle" and the big picture. Habitat and species loss are two other issues in nature that people ignore, and they go hand in hand.

We commit ourselves to "willful ignorance" about so many things. There is a reckoning coming. It's up to you and me and the truth we seek and the choices we make and the votes we cast. I don't want to be on the wrong side of history.

We are paying for our disregard. I grew up breaking ice in the winter in our frozen pond for our cattle to drink, but my 30-year-old daughter has never seen a frozen pond in the same part of the state. Sure, there are climate cycles; but there are other well-documented trends that scientists warned about for years way before anybody heard of Al Gore. Now, those warnings are becoming reality. People are being affected and endangered by those realities in more and more places.

I grew up watching the weather. In years past we didn't have natural disasters making the news almost every night. Now, we do. A study of statistics bears out that observation. Continuing to deny these realities is simply ignoring what is going on out there, being willfully ignorant of them, being isolated and unaware of them, and/or being untruthful. I cannot look myself, my God, and my grandchildren in the eye and not do my part to help.

Consider the costs of disregarding nature.

There are many "climate deniers" who think all this flurry about climate change, fossil fuels, regulations, policy change, and lifestyle change is the creation of "tree huggers," "butterfly chasers," and "manipulators" working in a conspiracy against business, progress, free enterprise, and even common-sense. Climate deniers speak of costs and bottom lines and being conservative. They ignore the insurance costs alone that are already hitting many of us because of weather changes connected to climate change—increased storms, flooding, and wildfires.

Just watch the news. Observe the increasing insurance issues all over America. Look at the battle over building and farming in floodplain areas and the insurability of all that. We can plan on seeing more of the same. It's high time we started caring about these superseding issues. They matter, and they've mattered for a long time. We cannot get away with environmental degradation forever. This may matter less to you than financial impacts, but we should all be saddened and spurred to action after the 2019 report that said we have lost 25 percent of our bird population (that's a loss of 3 billion birds) in the last 50 years. There's that much less tweeting outside your window. Take notice!

There are many places I could point you for more information. For example, Thomas Friedman's book *Hot, Flat, and Crowded* provides a truthful but hopeful perspective on these critical issues. Another source I'd point you to is the Nature Conservancy. I've donated to this organization for years and have kept up with its excellent conservation efforts and perspectives on environ-mental preservation. There is so much to become informed about, instead of being willfully misinformed or uninformed. Being unaware is still in vogue with many people. We need a change of perspective, and quick.

Our older daughter used to do the funniest thing when she was a toddler. If she was playing under, say, the dining room table and didn't want me to see her, she would sit up as high as possible. She thought that if we couldn't see her face, she was invisible. We'd laugh every time.

Lots of folks these days are participating in "willful ignorance" when it comes to the issues of nature. The times and the realities and the issues demand better of us. We need to read up, get informed, get in touch. What many folks are hearing from a "news source" with a well-funded agenda has become "reality" for them, but it's out of touch with reality and truth and science. Personally, I can do no less than become informed and act on the information I receive. I owe it to my family and to my God.

Vote your ethics.

Ethics deals with right and wrong, not just a "platform" that benefits you. Ethics inform commitments, and commitments determine choices and even lifestyles. If nothing changes in our heart or habits, what good is it?

A key time for being genuinely patriotic Americans is voting time. It's up to you and me to follow the news every day, pay attention to what leaders are saying and doing, and vote our conscience and ethics—informed conscience and ethics, not just "getting on the bandwagon" and its agenda. I've had to change many of the opinions I gained as I grew up. My observations, my learning, my heart, my faith: all these have demanded that I get on the right side of history.

Let your ethics and lifestyle match up.

It's so easy these days to get roped into the typical consumptive American lifestyle. But that lifestyle has consequences for our environment. It's up to you and me to learn about those things and make as many hard decisions as we can to alter our consumption. Those things affect the water, the air, the soil, plants and animals, and, yes, climate change.

What will you drive? How far will you commute, and how will you get there? How big does your home need to be? What water-saving practices could you implement? How do you vacation? How do you make your weekly buying choices as they relate to sustainability and environmental impact? How much do you recycle? These and other questions surround our ethical considerations about our natural world.

Immerse yourself in the natural world.

One of the most important ways to get in touch with our natural world is to get in it more. Step outside and linger in the early morning. Take in the rays of light through the trees. Watch the birds as they "work" your property. Step outside at sunset. Watch your daytime world pause for rest and watch the "night shift" emerge. Learn the daytime and nighttime creatures. Listen to their sounds. Let them be music to your ears. You may want to start at the bird feeders.

My wife and I have fed birds as long as we've been married. When our older daughter was just a tot of about 20 pounds, we began involving her in feeding and observing birds. She was serious about the "beefird," and would get quite a few chuckles at the grocery store when she insisted on carrying a 10-pound bag of beefird on her shoulder. Back home, she would be so cute as she helped me put out beefird, including several tiny little piles of seed that she would put on this rock and that stump, and show me each with pride. Both of our girls have come home from college telling funny stories about introducing friends on campus to "rufous-sided towhees" and "red-bellied woodpeckers" and on and on.

Beyond the bird feeders, there are many other things to discover. Foxes, possums, and raccoons delight young eyes. There's the beauty of each season—winter, spring, summer, and fall. There are unique parts of each of these seasons: snowfall in winter, flowers and baby birds in spring, young birds and animals that mature before our eyes over summer, and the quieter, subtler shades of all things that color the fall.

My wife and I have made many trips over the past 30 years with our girls (and now with our sons-in-law) where we've explored our North Georgia mountains, including part of the Appalachians. We've enjoyed imparting to our family an appreciation of millions of years of geologic time that have brought about the beauty before us, as well as the culture that has transpired over the region. Similarly, our trips to the Georgia coast have offered both a sense of history and an appreciation of the marshes and the coastal areas, the barrier islands and the ocean. These family discoveries—much more vivid in our minds than any putt-putt golf or shopping or "spectaculars" so common to American vacations—have enriched our lives, our memories, and our perspectives.

Revel in natural beauty.

There's nowhere I'd rather be than out in natural beauty. Over the years our family has enjoyed visiting beautiful places that have become dear to us, making many good memories. All of these trips were relatively inexpensive except one: our 1997 trip to Yellowstone National Park. In between the trips, we've reveled in natural beauty even right around us.

I love Northeast Georgia. I'm supremely happy when I'm there, and I always dislike leaving, even though I'm happy where we live and the life we have back home. I always tell folks how much I enjoy sitting on a rock in the middle of a mountain stream and watching and listening to the water flow over the rocks. Years spent visiting this region have afforded us wonderful experiences with family and friends, and an ever-increasing appreciation of its natural beauty, history, and culture. In contrast but equally wonderful are trips we've made to coastal areas.

Trips to Cumberland Island, for example, are memorable to us for the largely unchanged beauty of one of Georgia's barrier islands. On nearby Saint Simons Island, which is much more settled but still beautiful, I've enjoyed riding my bike from the south end to the north end and back, taking in the coastal beauty at a slower pace, vividly enjoying places such as the historic lighthouse, Fort Frederica, and Christ Church. I remember dodging a summer thunderstorm at Saint Simons and then pausing by a marsh area and observing birds, always with a little excitement at surprises before my eyes.

Though I've traveled my native state of Georgia extensively, and the South from Texas to West Virginia, and to Hawaii years ago, no "exotic" trip surpasses our trip to Yellowstone.

Visiting Yellowstone was a dream trip of a lifetime, a place I've studied for so long. It was everything I'd hoped for and more. Around every curve was incredible beauty and marvel. I'll never forget being at places including Old Faithful, the Falls of the Grand Canyon of the Yellowstone River, Mammoth Hot Springs, Yellowstone Lake, and, most of all, the incredible Lamar Valley. Seeing wildlife at so many turns was again and again such a delight. I do hope to return to Yellowstone someday and to explore it in more depth, especially since the reintroduction of wolves to the park.

The point here is to motivate you to learn to revel in the beauty of nature. It's wonderful beyond description to find great joys in nature, without waiting in line, without dressing to impress, without needing to shoot anything except photos, and sometimes almost without a sound.

Allow natural beauty to change you.

Discovering natural beauty without a need to compete within it or shoot it or beat it or fight it will change you. It will "tenderize" you and attune you to appreciate things more vividly. At the same time, discovering natural beauty will gradually "re-wild" you, making you more alert, more in touch with every sight and sound and smell around you, and just more in touch with the self you were created to be. If you've not been changed in these ways by the beauty of nature, then it's time to get out there and begin to let that happen.

Find out quickly what I'm talking about by stepping into nature's beauty and also by reading the classics of nature. Read Aldo Leopold's *Sand County Almanac*. If a person of faith, read the Green Bible. Read articles found in the *Nature Conservancy* social media pages. These can get you started and open doors to changing your perspective for the rest of your life.

Connect to nature through art and music.

The older I get, the more I'm drawn to the connection between nature and art and music. I love nature photography and paintings. I'm quite certain our little collection of nature art will continue to increase over the years, with a good story behind each piece. Music also connects with nature, both in its sounds and often poetic lyrics.

From hymns of faith such as "This Is My Father's World," to everyday songs such as the old Eddie Rabbitt hit "I Love A Rainy Night," to symphonic arrangements such as Aaron Copland's "Appalachian Spring" that capture some of the majesty of crashing oceans, peaceful sunrises, and flashing light-ning—all of these mediums offer a taste of nature when we're inside, exciting our memories, and driving us to get back outside again.

Find natural beauty in people.

I have a theory I bring up sometimes when people are talking about looks and beauty. I think almost everybody becomes beautiful when they become their authentic selves, when they become physically fit. Physical fitness brings out who you were created naturally to be. No makeup, plastic surgery, artifi-cial this or fake that, fancy shoes or nails or eyelashes or clothes or whatever are needed. It doesn't have to be something oversexed or creepy or lewd or anything like that, but in fact and indeed admirable. It's like taking a block of wood or clay and chipping away until all that remains is a beautiful sculpture. That's why fitness fascinates me so.

Physically at least, and, many of us would point out that mentally as well, fitness brings out the beauty in people naturally and at all ages. If we all could grasp this truth, many things about our world and our society would change.

If we could embrace this reality, our total health and psyche would change and become properly vibrant. Our relationships and lives would change.

Take care of yourself and be fully who you were created naturally to be.

*****

I hope I have motivated you to take care of yourself as you take care of nature. I hope you will move the needle in at least one or more ways to do something that changes our world for the better. I hope you will take actions to reduce your negative impact on nature, because most of us are impacting nature negatively every day. I hope you will get out and immerse yourself in nature now and regularly and always. "Immigrating inside" is damaging us in largely irreparable ways. While you're getting out and getting more into nature, take others along with you, especially children. The treasures you can discover are immeasurable.

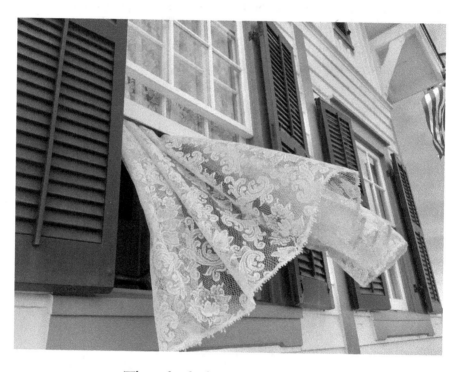

That ole clock never stops ticking.
Moments and opportunities slip by unnoticed.

Chapter 7

Take Care of Your Time and Interests

That ole clock never stops ticking. Moments and opportunities slip by unnoticed. Even if you are a busy, hardworking person, are you wasting time? Most of us have done it. I know I have. The older I get, the more I become aware of how precious is time. I've even learned that one of the most precious things we can give others is our time. We have to choose what we will do with each of those moments. Let's look at what we do with our time, interests, and energies and see if we can do better.

I love people, but many I meet are bored and/or boring. I pity some people for how little they have going on in their minds and in their lives. They make it obvious they're bored. I feel for them. Friends on Facebook, for example, share information that, if it's not angry, selfish, shortsighted political rants, it's mindless stuff about nothing. I'm not talking about people who have different interests from me. I'm talking about people who apparently have few interests in anything worthwhile or constructive.

Life is too short to live like that. There are so many things out there to find interest in and be involved in. Lots of folks have heard me say that I can't ever see me being bored. I have so much to do, so much to see, so much to read, not to mention bikes to ride, hikes to take, birds to watch, songs to sing, and cattle to tend. I'll never watch reruns of game shows all day!

Most weeks I encounter a number of people of all ages. I'm continually amazed at what I see out of their eyes: smiles, stress, anger, love, curiosity, sadness, excitement. Many of those eyes just reflect boredom—boredom with life, nowhere to go, nothing to be about, nothing on the mind, no twinkle in the eyes, living in a rut. We all need something to be about, even if it's just birds singing and the beauty of a sunset. I think a healthy curiosity may be one of the greatest gifts any of us can enjoy. Discover it. Cultivate it. Follow it. Enjoy it.

Examine what your "screen time" really means.

It seems that everybody's behind a screen these days, either on a smartphone or a tablet or a computer or a TV. Many of us are trying to fill a void by finding something on that screen. Some people are trying to gain or keep relationships through calling and texting and face-timing and hoping for Mr. or Mrs. Right through whatever app or site. Others are finding distraction through never-ending video games. These activities take up time, distract from the issues at hand, get our minds off things we'd rather not do or face. There's an endless array of things to find behind those screens, good and bad. How you handle them is all up to you. And, the results of those choices are, again, up to you.

Over the years I've noted what different people "follow" on social media such as Facebook, Twitter, or Instagram. A study of these habits reveals much about each of us and, behind that, the whys of it all. Maybe it's sports of all kinds. Maybe its casseroles and desserts. Maybe it's politics and political rants. But I always note the connection between what people "follow" and where they are emotionally, spiritually, and more.

What do you follow and why? What does that say about you? About what you fear? About what you're angry about and why? Or, maybe, hopefully, about what is good and kind and constructive and nourishing?

A lot of us need to take a long, hard look at what we're feasting on. I personally "follow" a lot of fitness, music, nature, cycling, waterfalls, cattle, and what I've deemed trustworthy news sources. Oh, and I do have a lot of "friends" of all sorts, and I do my best to be a friend as well.

So, how can we break out of the boredom? How can we overcome the mindless, corrosive addictions many of us are feeding on? How can we break the cycle?

Overcome disinterest; cultivate interests instead.

You'll be glad as you get older if you shake the boredom cycle now. Shake the corrosive "feeds" and addictions, and replace them with "whatever is good and true and beautiful," as the Bible tells us (Phil. 4:8). There are many wonderful things to focus on, study, be changed by, and contribute to. If you can be aware of and overcome the cynical, sarcastic, fearful, hateful, selfish forces so prevalent in society, you will have received a most wonderful gift. There are so many better, life-giving things out there to get wrapped up in.

The sky's the limit—there are so many choices. Many voices today are raising concern over "screen time" and "disconnection" and addiction to video games and other things we find on screens. But when we do have "screen time," there are many constructive things in which to engage.

Keep reading.

Step up your curiosity and regularly get a hold of stimulating and helpful things to read. These could be in books, magazines, or newspapers or on a screen or all of the above, but read, read, read. If you can read, doors open for you through the endless things you can learn.

I've read my way into more stuff than I can name. I spend much of my "non-moving" moments reading. I seem to especially love reading when eating out of a bowl. I don't know what that says about me, but there I am, eating my cereal or whatever, clinking my spoon, reading the news, social media, *Outside* magazine or *Nature Conservancy* magazine, or the latest book from my ever-growing stack.

Don't stop learning.

Unfortunately, many people stop learning after their last graduation. Maybe school took it all out of them. Maybe school taught them that learning is not fun. How unfortunate. It's up to you. You don't have to become nerdy, but learn something. Learn every day that you live. Get up and be alert to something you can learn. Never outlive your curiosity: it's so important to aging well.

The more I learn, the more I discover what I don't know. The more I learn, the more I want to learn. Learning opens a door that leads to another door, and another and another. Learning brings delight in new and wonderful discoveries. Learning offers greater gratitude as you discover how much there is for which to be thankful.

Observe with understanding and discernment.

If you learn that you don't know it all, then you have a chance to learn to understand and discern. Many of us just talk all the time without gaining understanding, and many of us feed off folks who talk all the time without understanding. We rush to judgment without discerning.

Perhaps our current times are what they are because of a rash of this phenomenon. One of the results of this problem is the lemming-like way in which many people join the crowd mentality and rush mindlessly off the cliff together. I see otherwise good people get duped and hoodwinked. Beware! Sometimes that learning curve is steep.

Don't waste your time; invest in it.

I joke with folks sometimes about how I wake up every morning still thinking in my mind that I'm a 16-year-old kid with brown hair. Then I step in front of the mirror and reality strikes. How did it happen overnight? How'd I get from my teens to my 50s? Where is time flying? Actually, I've been having a lot of fun much of this time. If it was all over today, I must say I've had a wonderful life with endless things for which I'm thankful. The older I get, the more I learn, the more I realize, the more I am aware of how precious is time.

Some people say nothing is more valuable than time. They wisely point out that when we boil down all the money we make, the accomplishments we consider so dear, the power and position and prominence we seek, when it's all over, we'll come out wishing we had much of that time back. Many of us would ask for a do-over. As one very old man said, he hopes his relatives won't talk about his bad stuff when he's gone but will instead focus on what he did that was good.

The clock is ticking incessantly for each of us. None of us are getting any younger. As some say, none of us will get out alive. Time is such a precious commodity. Carpe diem! Make every day count. Savor the moments.

If you've already graduated from high school, recall the graduation speeches you heard. Many graduation speakers use the phrase, "as we stand here on the threshold of life." It's a true phrase, but I admit it does make me grin. Graduation really is a threshold to the rest of your life. It's not a trite nothing when we urge people to not live a life wasted.

The Eagles have long been one of my favorite singing groups. I've always loved the line in their song, "Take It to the Limit," that says "You can spend all your time making money; you can spend all your life making time." Don't run out the clock and have nothing lasting to show for your time. Don't live a life wasted. Be about something, and be about something truly good.

Live with purpose.

Purposeful living makes even downtime more fulfilling. Please don't hear me saying you always need to be doing something. Sometimes you need to just lie in the grass and stare up at the sky. With all the balance I'm advocating in this book, I surely don't want to assert that we should be Type AAA people who can never relax and must "make every minute count." Downtime is essential to good mental, spiritual, relational, and physical health.

Downtime, rest, and relaxation are part of the rhythm of life. Making the most of our days and not wasting our time and our lives make "respite" periods more satisfying. It's then that we can best savor what we've accomplished, experienced, and learned, and also the many good things that happen in our lives. We need time to rest, recover, recreate, relax, ponder, worship, and more. Find this rhythm between action and inaction—the balance that brings satisfaction to your life.

Purposeful living should define our occupations and preoccupations: What if our jobs were not just about the grind and making money? What if we actually enjoyed our jobs? What if we found fulfillment while doing our jobs?

The good news is that many of us know these joys. The bad news is that many of us hate our jobs and everything about them. The great news is that sometimes our skills, needs, and what gives us joy and what makes a suitable living financially all come together. If we worked our economy smarter and if we guided young people more deliberately, we'd have better matches of purpose, giftedness, joy, and higher pay.

I hope to retire someday; in fact, I'm working toward it with the help of my financial planner. Most folks I know intend to retire at some point, too. What we will do when we retire varies considerably, however.

When I listen to people's retirement plans, and when I watch what they do in retirement, it's obvious that my retirement plans are different. Maybe my most famous retirement "model" is former President Jimmy Carter. In his mid-90s, when I read about what he's done lately, he makes me feel lazy.

I have all sorts of things in mind for when I retire. I'll volunteer and sing at my church. I'll volunteer with a couple of nature organizations. Oh, I'll probably stick my nose into area and regional planning meetings. I'll keep exercising, riding bikes, hiking to waterfalls, tending my cows and my garden, birdwatching, reading, writing, and most of all spending time with family and friends. How could I ever be bored? Sound like your retirement plans?

Rest and relax without "grinding" about doing something.

Can you never really be at ease? Have you been identified as Type A? I know and love so many Type A's and Type AAA's. They're get-things-done kinds of people. They're high achievers. On the other hand, on those personality tests I've scored Type B every time. I've worked hard all of my life. I've been involved in all sorts of things. Many times I've been too involved and too busy, but I've never had a hard time relaxing and resting.

I can sit on a porch and watch sunsets. Never does a day pass that I'm not watching birds at least for a few moments. I sing along with something every day. I can enjoy a restful holiday or weekend break. I don't always have to be overachieving or plotting how to beat my competitor. It appears that I'm succeeding at worrying less and less as I get older.

How about you? Do you long to be "off," then can't be off when you're off? Are you too serious? What do the kids in your life say about that? Are they right? Again, being able to find balance and get in sync with the natural rhythm of life can be hard for many of us. Master the art!

Be present with people who matter, and others who should.

Sometimes we're not really present with people even when we're with them. We're there in body but not in mind and spirit; our mind is somewhere else. This is especially true in the day of the ubiquitous smartphone. Ever almost been hit by a car while walking and looking at your cellphone? Ever spent a weekend with someone who had their nose in their cellphone the whole time?

Screen addictions or not, it is well documented and in fact commonsense that our relationships will be enriched if we will offer each other the courtesy of being present when we are present. Now, there are times when I have to take a moment and handle something on my smartphone or take care of business while in the midst of other people. But I try to apologize and then step away. Sometimes, though, I make it all wait and just stay tuned to who's in front of me. Do you have trouble with that? There may be a beautiful woman trying to get your attention. There may be people behind you in line who wish you would move ahead. There may be something else you need to discover right under your nose.

Way before there were smartphones and tablets and video games to hypnotize us, there were other distractions. I vividly remember a 12-year-old boy I used to be around. He so badly wanted some attention out of his bored and distracted dad. He told me it seemed about the only thing he ever saw of his dad was two hands holding a newspaper. That dad stayed engaged with something else all the time, but not with the boy.

Our kids need us to show something to live for. Our spouses need us to remember the spirit in which we married, why we were in love, why we were fascinated with each other. Pay attention! Come out from behind the screen, the newspaper, the façade, the cloud of anger, the busyness, the bottle, whatever it is, and be present with people who matter—and maybe also with the people who you need to realize matter. Wake up! Life is in front of you and all around you. Engage!

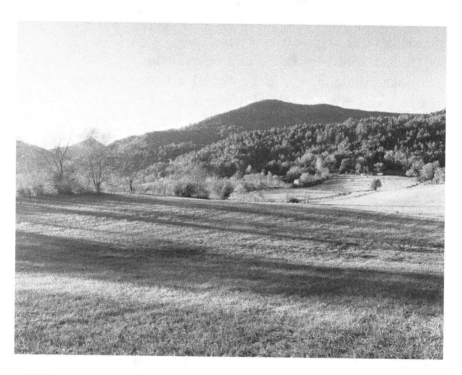

What you enter this world with and what you leave this world with are the same except for who you love, the memories you enjoy, the contributions you make, and the character you become.

Epilogue

I've tried to share so much in this book—maybe too much, but I want to help you take care of yourself. Look through these pages and see what could help you. Take care of yourself, both now and as long as you live. You'll be glad you did, and the sooner the better. There are endless reasons to take care of yourself. Maybe I've lived longer than you have. Maybe I'm 30 years younger than you. Either way, let's look at some highlights of why you should take care of yourself now and tomorrow.

Take care of your body now and always.

Do something every day to make things better for yourself and your body. If you aren't getting stronger and fitter, you're losing ground. Add that up over time, and the effects get exponential. And quit telling yourself that taking care of your body doesn't matter. It does. Quit telling yourself that you'll take care of your body tomorrow or next week or next year. No, now's the time! You're precious and your body is precious. It's not about vanity, but hey, maybe you'll look a little better. You'll like that. You'll be happier with yourself. Get going.

Take care of your mind, spirit, and emotions.

A healthier mind, spirit, and emotions can help the health of your body, and taking care of your body reciprocally helps your mind, spirit, and emotions. There are many things we could do to think better thoughts, to have a more vibrant spirit and deeper spirituality, and to have more stable, happy, and caring emotions. Now's the time to heal. Now's the time to set a course for a freer and healthier spirit. Now's the time to start going deeper in your faith. Now's the time to stop "flapping in the wind," to stop being buffeted by every wind gust and every whim, and to become "unflappable." There's so much to discover and gain in the realm of your mind, spirit, and emotions.

Take care of your relationships.

Who you love should be a big deal to you. If you're lonely, get a handle on the reasons. Maybe you're loved more than you know. Maybe you've forsaken your relationships for interests you've mistakenly put ahead of them. Your relationships truly are your most precious "possessions." Actually, your relationship with yourself is affected and colored by all the aspects detailed in this book. This is personal!

Take care of your community.

Truly, "no man is an island." And, honestly, no one is completely "self-made." We each live in context, in community. Your place is more important than what you can get out of it. There's also what you need to put back into it. As you "bloom where you're planted," it's important to be aware of where that is and all the seen and unseen connections to you there.

Take care of your things.

Your things define you more than you realize or admit. Stuff is a huge factor in most of our daily lives. Nowadays we relate to stuff differently and in degrees never before seen by any other society. Your relationship to and your ideas and activities about things determine much about you.

Take care of your world.

You still may not realize what a precious world you've been born into. You may yet have much to discover and appreciate about our world and about nature. I hope this book has awakened your awareness to nature and will spur you to get involved in protecting it.

Take care of your time and interests.

Will you ever be bored again? Probably. I hope I've given you some pointers that could help you develop curiosities and invest your time well. Life is too wonderful to pass through it unexplored, unquestioned, unimpressed, just marking time. Wake up!

*****

I come from a particular corner of mainstream Christianity. I do not relate to much of what I've seen coming out of popular Christianity over the last 40 years. That said, I wish to share here my take on biblical and theological foundations for taking care of yourself. I hope you'll find them helpful, as they have been for me.

Taking care of yourself, beyond being a benefit to yourself, is an act of appreciation for what your Creator has given you. Genesis 1:27 states that God created us in the image of God. So many things are implied here, but one thing I take away from it is that we are dear to God, valued immensely by God, and therefore we should appreciate all that we've been given. This should make us want to take care of ourselves as an act of gratitude and stewardship.

We are all the aspects of our personhood combined. They all matter, so we shouldn't tend to one aspect and neglect another. Some people seek to tend to the spiritual aspects of personhood and neglect their body. Others do the opposite. I'm convinced God wants us to keep everything in balance and to take care of ourselves in all the ways I've detailed. There is no reason to neglect one area to take care of another. Balance is the key.

Taking care of your body should be as important spiritually as any other aspect of your being. I find a number of scriptures that point to caring for our bodies, but perhaps none more clearly than 1 Corinthians 6:19-20 that tells us our body is a temple of the Holy Spirit. It says we belong to God and that we should honor God with our body. Many Christians emphasize shortsightedly that this means we must not engage in improper sexual activities. I would point out that, in addition to sexual ethics, this teaching points to honoring God by the care we give our bodies.

Many of us have a limited theology of the body and its care and aesthetics, and indeed our sexual ethics and attitudes. There's way too much awkwardness about bodies and how we act toward each other. While we fight over and scream over and try to ignore the #MeToo Movement, we ignore thousands of years of men and women abusing each other and going about things so wrongly. We ought to be able to handle all these sexual and relational dynamics with greater maturity and awareness. Just because we see a beautiful car doesn't mean we have to drive it or steal it or beat it up. Just because we see someone who is attractive doesn't mean we have to pursue, harass, ogle, or speak lewdly toward or about that person. We need to grow up! We need to be aware of powerful dynamics that can go on between people, and apply wisdom to those interactions.

When it comes to the care of our own bodies, I think it is evident that we would glorify God and show appreciation to God much more if we would give our bodies the best of care and fitness, instead of the neglect that probably 99 percent of us do. Care of our bodies, along with proper behavior and ethics among us, would be more in line with a good theology of our body.

Taking care of our mind, spirit, and emotions is another aspect of selfhood that needs greater religious, spiritual, and theological understanding. Mark 12:28-31 perhaps gives the ultimate instruction, in fact, surely the most important instruction of Jesus Christ, speaking to all situations we face. This "greatest commandment" tells us how we should love God with all our heart, all our soul, all our mind, and all our strength. We should love God by how we care for and present our body, by how we use our mind (no closed minds, no dumbing down, for example), by devoting our spirituality in the most fervent ways, and by allowing our heart to be expanded again and again as we find more ways to love and understand and give.

There are countless ways we can explore and apply the greatest commandment within ourselves and with all those around us. While we're living out these teachings, our emotions can take on a more beautiful character. We can become less reactive and more responsive. We can gain more hope and overcome hopelessness. We can see possibilities and overpower cynicism. We can choke out reckless anger as we cultivate overwhelming love. It's all a lifetime growth process.

While we're on the greatest commandment passage, we get the directive we need for taking care of our relationships: "Love your neighbor as you love yourself" (Mark 12:31). Well, that'll require some changes from us. I cross paths with a lot of people in an average week. Some of them are real treasures; some of them are not. More and more, as I meet strange or rude or different people in, say, the grocery store, just as my ridicule starts up, a voice inside me reminds me that, hey, Jesus loves them too. It changes how I regard these people.

Whether you are a devotee to Christianity or not, I wish more of us, believers or not, could discover that it is first and foremost a religion of love. Most of us have obviously forsaken that message. All our relationships are affected by our understanding or misunderstanding of love and all its demands and applications. Taking care of our relationships calls forth this and all the other teachings on love.

When we reach beyond ourselves, we immediately reach into our community. In taking care of ourselves, we do well if we contribute to taking care of our community. This principle is central in Christian teachings, yet neglected and misunderstood by most modern Christians. Instead of making us more smug, fearful and defensive, the focus should be outward and redemptive and reconciling.

To me, no passage is clearer about this than 2 Corinthians 5:19, emphasizing that, in Christ, God was reconciling the world to himself. Most Christians stop right there in their understanding, outlook, and practice. But there's more to it. It goes on to say that God has committed to us the message of reconciliation. If we take this seriously, it will change many of the "mission" activities of our churches. It will challenge our attitudes about people and society. It may even change our politics. It will require us to "question everything and hold on to the good" (1 Thess. 5:20-22). It will move us to become involved in bringing greater good to our community, our town, our county, our state, our nation, our world. It will demand more of us than we'd thought about.

Taking care of ourselves includes taking care of our things. Jesus had more to say about our possessions than most of us find comfortable. This reality should affect what we possess and how we use and care for our possessions. Jesus urged that we "not store up treasures on earth" that are subject to being destroyed or stolen, but instead we should "store up treasures in heaven" (Matt. 6:19).

One verse really isn't enough to fully inform us, and one verse isn't enough to challenge our attitudes and addictions with our stuff. Another verse that illustrates the attitude and mindset of Jesus is his directive to travel lightly (Luke 9:3). Moving past a shortsighted, legalistic interpretation of this passage, we take note of the entire story of Jesus—he had disregard and even disdain for all our "stuff." What would he say to us now, the way most of us live?

Every year at Christmas, in the midst of all the celebrating I so enjoy, I also ponder how disdained Jesus surely is about all the junk that will be unwrapped in his name, at how the landfills will swell on this day, how so many of us worried and rushed and literally fought over stuff in stores, and our attitudes about all of that.

Taking care of our world has close ties to the width and breadth of Scripture. In biblical times, not unlike how most of our ancestors lived up until World War II, people were much more closely tied to the earth and the things of the earth. When Jesus spoke of fishing or farming, the people of his day knew exactly what he was talking about. The parables were not as foreign to them as to us. People nowadays think milk comes from the store and water comes from a faucet. The Old Testament, however, is laced with references from where it all came.

Beyond the Creation accounts in Genesis, for example, I think of Psalm 19:1 that points out "the heavens are telling the glory of God." I first came to love this passage put to music when in high school I got to sing with our chorus' performance of Haydn's "The Heavens Are Telling." I cannot hear this verse without hearing the majestic first chords of this piece. Another favorite of mine and countless others is Psalm 23. This heartwarming poem of devotion speaks of shepherds, sheep, green pastures, still waters—an idyllic and peaceful picture. Even in dark valleys, a warm intimacy with our Creator and Sustainer is envisioned and assured. It is from these passages and many others that we can undeniably come to a biblical and Christian ethic of environmental responsibility and stewardship.

Iconic theologian Glenn Hinson in his book, *The Reaffirmation of Prayer*, speaks of "the distance we have put between ourselves and nature. In conquering nature, we have denatured ourselves. We have suppressed some natural and instinctive responses, among which may be the restlessness of a heart which seeks God." From this and other points, Dr. Hinson, and I, would point out that so much of our unnatural and destructive lifestyle forces are in part our efforts to fill voids in our lives caused by our disconnect from our natural and earthy world. These are just some of the reasons we seek fulfillment in buying more things— and in digging inexplicably in the refrigerator and pantry late at night.

Taking care of ourselves as we take care of our time and interests has plenty of directives in Scripture, starting in the first verses of Genesis. God created the heavens, the earth, day, night, plants, birds, animals . . . and it was very good—so much to get up for every day, no time to waste. Am I waxing poetic, or am I on to something? Maybe our time and even our curiosity are gifts to be maximized.

In Psalm 102 we read: "My days are like the evening shadow; I wither away like grass" (v. 11). So quickly it all passes by. Repeatedly, the Scriptures teach us to make the most of our days, to be about doing something good and helpful in our needy world.

Are you wasting your time, your mind, your curiosities, and your abilities? Are time, teaching, training, and talents wasted on you? Are you frittering it all away?

I've seen too many people squander their lives away—so much wasted time. I don't want to do that. And, I react in dread at the thought of rotting away in boredom. Every time we exclaim "Why doesn't *somebody* do something about . . .?" the answer comes bouncing back from God like an echo in a canyon: Why don't *you* do something about it? Scripture teaches us that God gives us the time, abilities, and impetus to move out and do something worthwhile in our needy, tormented world. It's time to get going!

*****

The fall of 2017 brought a lot to deal with in my life. It had been a normally busy year in my real estate world and with all my other involvements. The second week of September, in Georgia we were hunkering down as Hurricane Irma was making its way inland as a tropical storm, with lots of wind and rain. I got a call that morning that my dad had fallen and was taken to the hospital. I began making my way across Atlanta in stormy conditions to see about him.

First results were that he was just banged up again from yet another fall, so we took him home. We still had a few questions, especially about his right foot pointing too far to the right. A few days later a second check revealed he had a broken hip. That weekend he would have extensive hip surgery. This had been quite a blow to him and to our family. Things would no longer be the same for him, in a number of ways. I would be back and forth with my folks a lot as the days went on, seeing after their care, but otherwise all was normal. Then my turn came in October.

It was my 55th year, and I worked into my calendar a normally scheduled colonoscopy. Due to double family history, I'd been having that procedure at predetermined times since my late 30s. Things had always gone well. I had continued to work at taking care of myself, dialing in my diet and exercise to the best level of my adult life. I felt as good as I had in years, maybe ever. Then I got a call.

My longtime gastroenterologist wanted me to come in and consult regarding results of the colonoscopy. I was driving around when I took the call, and was immediately concerned. I asked when was the soonest I could get an appointment. There was one left that day in the late afternoon. "I'll take it!"

My wife joined me for the appointment. The doctor shared with us in a very serious tone that an area of rough texture had been noted in my colon and that needle biopsies had revealed mantle cell lymphoma, a non-Hodgkin's lymphoma. He had already consulted initially with an oncologist at the hospital, shared the good news that this was minuscule and found very early, and that they had a treatment plan in mind that would have me in remission in the spring. Still, it was serious stuff. I had never faced anything like this.

Treatment and recovery went as the medical personnel had forecasted. After being diagnosed in October, and after weeks of tests and preparation and consultations, I started rounds of chemo in December. After wonderful care by doctors and nurses at Piedmont Fayette Hospital and Northside Hospital in Atlanta, after seven rounds of chemo and the removal and reintroduction of my stem cells, after weeks of post-stem cell and other follow-up treatments, and after completing 100 days of quarantine, I was declared to be in remission. I carefully rejoined society while continuing follow-up and immunotherapy treatments. In light of all that I've experienced, it's beyond words for me to begin to describe how thankful I am and how wonderful things are now. So, here are some things I tell folks all the time:

I cannot ever thank my lovely wife enough for how she cared for me through it all. In addition to her faithfulness to me, she's the busy CFO of her commercial construction company, plus all the other realms of life we find ourselves in. I tell folks she proved to be a "magician," driving me back and forth for countless appointments and treatments, moving with me to Atlanta's north side for more than a month's time in an extended-stay suite near the second hospital, all the while magically working remotely on her laptop for hours each day doing her CFO work. She made it all happen, without complaining, and still being her beautiful self as always. She was never bedraggled and struggling. We laughed more than you would believe, and we got through the struggle of it all in surprisingly good fashion. We never had a tense word between us.

Giving thanks was and is my first response in the face of my cancer diagnosis—not for it, but in it. Getting a diagnosis of any kind of cancer is not something to be thankful about. But one of the first things I did at length after being told this bad news was to give thanks. First, I was thankful for a good diagnosis. I was thankful that my long-time gastroenterologist had gone ahead and consulted with a trusted oncologist in the hospital about my case. I was thankful that these doctors had at least an initial plan, which predicted I would be in remission in a few months.

Second, and overarching, I immediately shared with my wife my perspective of how much for which I was thankful—especially the life I've known with her and our family and closest friends. I expressed the vivid awareness I already had of how fortunate I am. I said that, regardless of the outcome, I would win. I meant it. I wasn't trying to be poetic or religious or heroic or to prop her up by being fluffy. I fully believed that, and I still do.

I committed myself to having bad days only one time. I articulated to my wife that I wouldn't "preload" my bad days. I wouldn't sit and worry and agonize and overthink and obsess over what could come. On my bad days I surprised myself at how much I followed that commitment. I've known times in my life when I could overthink with the best of them. The last few years I've really learned and assimilated some of the lessons about stress that I've shared earlier in this book. And I proved those lessons true once again "in the clutch time."

IRREPRESSIBLE! For me it meant unstoppable, can't keep me down, can't put a lid on me. In sharing this thought with a couple of friends, I said if you put a lid on me, a hand will come creeping out and then the rest of me. I was determined to be irrepressible. It's a good outlook for the trials of life.

Bad days come, but we don't need to live them twice. Take them when they come, but don't sit and ruin another day imagining what they might be like. If you follow that rule, you'll have fewer bad days and you'll be stronger when they come. Get your checkups on time, and be as strong and healthy as you can be. Whatever you're supposed to be checked for, get it done and on time. And, *take care of yourself.* Now, let's explore further these tips.

If I'd put off my scheduled colonoscopy for three years, until age 55, I either wouldn't have been around anymore or the disease would have been much more advanced. There are various screenings we all can be advised to have at different times, depending on individual and family history. It is advisable to adhere to these. My experience bears that out. Also, make the effort, invest the discipline, wise up, and take care of yourself. Become the fittest you can be and keep it up for the rest of your life.

Being as fit and strong as you can be is not a punishment or drudgery. It can be a joy to eat well and get regular exercise. If you think otherwise, you simply haven't tried the right things yet. The hopes of all that I'm advising here is that you'll never need it, that you'll pass away in your sleep at 98 after a wonderful, healthy, happy life. But both medical science and my own experience bear out the truth that getting checkups on time are for your advantage.

Also, being as healthy and fit as you can be will enrich your life and work to your advantage if some health malady does arise. That is my experience and is what medical personnel told me was the case countless times during my bout with cancer. They told me that my condition at the time of my diagnosis helped me recover more easily and quickly. Thankfully, I had "a lot of stock to burn up" during the travails of treatment and recovery. It took me a long way down. I maintained as much activity as was allowed and that I could muster, even during my worst days. I remember doing yard work during the winter even the next day after chemo. Later, I would reach a stage where I was restricted from doing yard work and other activities for a number of reasons. Still, I continued with walking and other activities as allowed (and encouraged) immediately after the last and harshest round of chemo and after stem cell replacement. I returned to basic exercises and to bike rides as soon as my doctors okayed it. All these things have aided my recovery. Get moving and stay moving!

I credit my cycling experiences with giving me extra grit and determination that helped me endure the cancer treatment and recovery process. Over the years I've had countless days and nights of fun, exciting, refreshing cycling experiences, both on-road and off-road, in five states, in all sorts of weather and temperatures (from the 20s to 100-plus degrees), in the rolling hills where I've spent most of my life, but also in my favorite mountains and on the flats along the coast. I'm always ready for the next ride. But among all those experiences, I can detail a number of times when I've had to dig deep to make it through and to return to my home base.

There have been times when I was riding while sick or not feeling well. I recall a few years ago when I took a couple of my cousins mountain biking by Tallulah Gorge in the North Georgia mountains, my favorite corner of the world. I hadn't had an asthma spell in more than 10 years, then one hit that very day, just for the day. I was chugging the whole ride, but I was glad I pressed on. Still, it afforded great moments with my cousins.

Several years earlier I embarked on my longest group ride so far: 115 miles in one day, from Peachtree City to Pine Mountain/Callaway Gardens to Warm Springs and back. What a fascinating trip! The camaraderie and the scenery and the challenge—I did well . . . until I enjoyed some red velvet cake at our lunch stop at the Bulloch House, a long-time favorite in Warm Springs. As I've since learned, cake is not good ride fuel. I felt like I was going to have a baby (OK, I really don't know what that feels like). I felt bad, with many hot miles to go. I pressed on, slower than I wanted, but digging deep and grinding it out, mile after mile.

I can think of many other times, in various weather and various situations, when I was having "a bad day"—but as we bikers say, a bad day on the bike beats all sorts of things. I realized numerous times during my cancer treatment and recovery journey how much all that "digging deep" had prepared and helped me to endure.

In addition to cycling, music and singing are a big part of my life. Mention about anything to me and a song lyric will come up. When people talk about how to live, "Wasted Days and Wasted Nights" by Freddy Fender and the Eagles' "Wasted Time" spring to mind.

No matter your age, time is precious. Don't waste it. Live life to the fullest. Make the most of your days. Live like you don't know how long you've got. And, take care of yourself. It's too easy to squander your life, your time, your money, your interests, your relationships, and more with activities and people that waste your time. Set out now to not live that way. Be thoughtful about what you engage in. Be choosy about what you devote yourself to. Ask: "Where is this going? Where is this taking me?" You'll be glad and thankful if you spend your days doing those things and being involved with those people and causes that bring lasting satisfaction.

As you live your precious moments, in all aspects of life, take care of yourself. And, as you do that, you'll take care of others and our world. Now, get going.

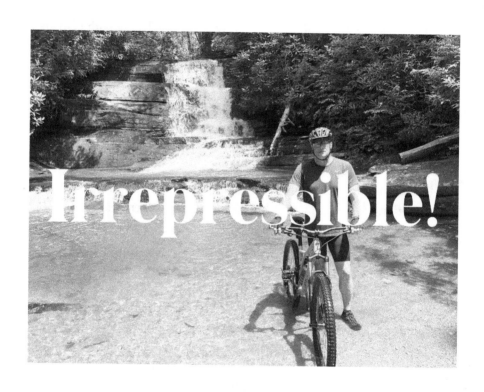

Irrepressible!